Comments on **Epilepsy at your** *your* 's

'I know that the book will be o. y
and their families.'
Joan Gorton, Honorary Se -p

'The text is clear and covers many _ manner.'
Monica Cooper, Man _formation Centre,
_ish Epilepsy Association

Epilepsy at your fingertips

The comprehensive and medically accurate
manual which tells you how to deal with
epilepsy with confidence!

Brian Chappell BEd
*National Manager, Neuroeducation, Department of Neurosciences,
York District Hospital; former Director of Information and Training,
British Epilepsy Association*

Dr Pamela Crawford MB ChB MD FRCP
*Consultant Neurologist, Director of the Special Centre for Epilepsy,
Department of Neurosciences, York District Hospital; Visiting Professor
of Community Neurological Studies, Leeds Metropolitan University*

CLASS PUBLISHING · LONDON

This book has been developed from *Your child's epilepsy: a parent's guide*,
written by Dr Richard Appleton, Brian Chappell and Margaret Beirne.

The charter for people with epilepsy is the copyright of the British Epilepsy
Association and has been reprinted with their kind permission.

The authors and publishers welcome feedback from the users of this book.
Please contact the publishers.

Class Publishing (London) Ltd, Barb House, Barb Mews, London W6 7PA
Telephone: 0171 371 2119
Fax: 0171 371 2878 [International +44171]
email: post@class.co.uk
Website: http://www.class.co.uk

A CIP catalogue record for this book is available from the British Library

ISBN 1 872362 51 6

Designed by Wendy Bann

Edited by Michèle Clarke

Indexed by Val Elliston

Cartoons by Jane Taylor

Line illustrations by David Woodroffe

Production by Landmark Production Consultants Ltd, Princes Risborough

Typesetting by DP Photosetting, Aylesbury, Bucks

Printed and bound in Finland by WSOY

02 01 00 99   10 9 8 7 6 5 4 3 2

Contents

Contents

Acknowledgements

We are grateful to anyone who has made a contribution, however small, to this book. In particular we should like to thank the following people for their contributions and support:

Dr Richard Appleton and Margaret Beirne who, with Brian Chappell, wrote a previous book for parents of children with epilepsy – their original research and text made this book for adults so much easier to write, saving an incalculable amount of time;

Avril Stewart, for her continuing help and advice;

the National Information Centre staff at the British Epilepsy Association for collecting most of the original questions;

Joan Gorton, Alison Iliff and Monica Cooper for helping with further questions and reviewing the manuscript;

all the people at Class Publishing who have helped us keep to the straight and narrow, Jane Taylor for her charming mouse cartoons and David Woodroffe for his illustrations.

Lastly, but certainly not least, we should like to thank the people with epilepsy who contributed their personal feelings for the section 'My Epilepsy'.

Foreword

by Sir ROBIN DAY

To see, as I have done, someone you know and love – someone
who is otherwise normal and healthy – having an epileptic seizure,
is an experience that can make a spectator feel bewildered,
frightened and helpless.

Epilepsy has been known for centuries, with records in the
Bible and pyramids, but still too little is known about this condition, its causes and its treatment.

Epilepsy can develop in anyone, at any age, but especially in
childhood, adolescence and old age. At least half a million people
in the UK have epilepsy. Many of them are children or teenagers.
On a child, and on the family of that child, the effects of epilepsy
can be devastating. Seizures may cause social rejection and isolation. Those affected by epilepsy, especially children at school,
may encounter ignorance, fear and prejudice.

Epilepsy is the most common brain disorder in the world. It has
also been one of the most overlooked and neglected of all medical
problems. Fortunately seizures can now often be controlled by
medication, but some epilepsies – about 20% – are extremely
resistant to drug treatment. Recent research gives hope that new
drug therapies are being developed that could transform the lives
of sufferers.

Sometimes the cause of epilepsy is unknown. Sometimes it is
caused by an accident, such as a serious head injury. Some people
are born with epilepsy. Much progress has been made by research
into the causes of epilepsy and its treatment, but epilepsy is not a
'headline' condition like cancer, AIDS and multiple sclerosis. So

much more information and advice is needed about how to help people who suffer from epilepsy.

Hence the great value of this book *Epilepsy at your fingertips*. Its authors are distinguished specialists in the study and treatment of epilepsy. They give expert answers to the questions which, in their experience, worry or puzzle people about epilepsy.

Foreword

by Dr STEPHEN BROWN FRCPsych

Consultant Neuropsychiatrist, Norwich Community Health Partnership NHS
Trust & Honorary Senior Lecturer, University of East Anglia School of Health;
Chair, Epilepsy Task Force, Formerly Chair, British Epilepsy Association

People often feel that doctors are rushed when they see them at
the hospital, and that there isn't time to ask questions. An
appointment with the doctor is also often an event that makes
people anxious, and may not be the best time to talk things over.
Yet it is important that people with epilepsy, and their friends and
families, are able to find out as much as they want to about the
condition. When we ask people with epilepsy, they nearly always
tell us that they wish they were given more information.

Every day in the United Kingdom more than 100 people are told
that they have epilepsy. In the majority of cases good treatment
will ensure that seizures are controlled. However, many people
with epilepsy face problems stemming from well-intentioned
overprotection and restriction of opportunity, for there are many
myths surrounding the condition, which can affect everyday life.
These might be overcome if the proper facts were more widely
known. Also, people who still have seizures would find it helpful
to know the full range of treatments available, so that they may
engage in an informed dialogue with their doctors.

Combining ease of reading with depth of information, Brian
Chappell and Pamela Crawford have ensured that readers won't
be intimidated by this book and that the information is easy to
locate with a simple question and answer approach. There is much
practical advice about everyday life, as well as a clear description
of important medical facts. This book should therefore play an
important part in helping people living with epilepsy, their families

and friends, in understanding the condition, and its impact on their lives.

Stephen Brown

The Charter for people with epilepsy

The British Epilepsy Association believes that people with epilepsy:

- are individuals and should be respected and treated as such;

- should be offered education and training opportunities in the community to suit their needs and abilities;

- are entitled to employment policies and procedures based on their skills, experience and qualifications;

- sometimes have particular needs which should be met by a system of disability benefits and allowances;

- deserve quality medical care from practitioners who understand epilepsy, on a free and accessible basis;

- have the right to information to help them choose whether or not to undergo any treatment offered;

- should be able to say 'I have epilepsy' without being rejected or labelled by others.

Introduction

To be told that you have epilepsy can be a shocking or even traumatic experience. Faced with this news, most people are anxious to obtain all the facts and to learn as much about epilepsy as they possibly can. A great deal of information is already available in various formats – medical textbooks, books, leaflets, videos, audiocassettes, even computer packages. There are also various epilepsy associations which can provide help, advice and information. So why, with all this information available, is there a need for another book on the subject?

Above all, we felt that people with epilepsy deserved a book which was written especially for them. We have tried to cover all aspects including the obvious medical issues, e.g. the different types of epilepsy and the different treatments available. There are many questions on the important issues, e.g. employment, drugs, pregnancy and contraception, other people's attitudes to epilepsy and leisure activities.

What about the other obvious sources of information – for example, the doctors who are looking after your epilepsy? Doctors and other health professionals are seen by many as the 'experts', and certainly they have an important role to play in helping to ensure successful medical treatment. However, it is unfortunate, but understandable, that not every doctor has specialist knowledge about epilepsy, and some people may therefore experience some difficulty in obtaining all the information that they would like to have. Fear of 'wasting the doctor's time' may mean that we are reluctant to ask questions, or to ask for an answer to be explained in more detail, or to ask for information to be repeated, although none of these things is time-wasting. Even when a lot of facts about epilepsy are provided, you may still be unclear as to whether all these facts apply to your own condition. Some questions may not be answered, whatever your source of information.

Medical advances happen all the time and some of these advances will make things easier for people with epilepsy, but we are not yet in sight of a cure or a 'magic' pill which will solve everyone's problems. Certainly a change in society's attitude to epilepsy could – and would – make many people's lives easier. As with so many things in life, it is you and your family who can make the most difference. We hope that this book will provide you with some ideas and help while you are trying to find out more about epilepsy, that you will also find it useful and informative, and that it will answer some, or even most, of the questions that you wanted to ask.

How to use this book

Because different people will have different requirements for information about their epilepsy, this book has been designed in such a way that you do not have to read it from cover to cover, unless you wish to do so. Instead it can be used selectively to meet your own particular needs. The questions are arranged into chapters and sections, so you may prefer to dip into the book a section at a time, or to look for information on a particular topic by using the contents list and the index. Cross-references in the answers will lead you to more detailed information where this might be helpful, and essential information is repeated whenever it seems to be necessary.

The first part of the book covers the medical management of epilepsy, while the second covers its social management. We have tried to treat these equally, as they are both extremely important and are frequently interlinked. When epilepsy first presents itself, it is usually seen as a medical issue: after all, your first contact is with a doctor. However, it soon becomes apparent that social issues are just as important, and that epilepsy cannot be managed completely successfully without addressing or dealing with both areas.

Not everyone will agree with every answer that we have given, but future editions of this book can only be improved by feedback from the people who know most about living with epilepsy – in other words, you. If you have any comments about the book, we would be delighted to receive them. It is also very important for us to know of any questions that have not been asked in this book, or of any other topics that you think should have been covered. Please write to us c/o Class Publishing, Barb House, Barb Mews, London W6 7PA.

What we have not done in this book is to tell you what it feels like to have epilepsy. That information can only come from people with personal experience, and so we have asked five of them to contribute their own accounts – these are given on the following pages. All the various types of epilepsy that they mention are discussed in detail elsewhere in the book.

My Epilepsy

From Arsène, a 34-year-old with epilepsy

I developed epilepsy as a result of an illness when I was $2\frac{1}{2}$, which has meant that I have had little choice but to come to terms with it and cope with it. Coming from a family background of doctors, I was fortunate enough that my epilepsy was diagnosed very quickly.

I believe that both my parents overplayed my early achievements in front of their friends because of my epilepsy, but thankfully, they never prevented me from swimming or cycling, both of which I loved and they encouraged.

Although I have never experienced the shock of being told that I had epilepsy, I have experienced on several occasions the distress that people have endured after being diagnosed with the condition in later life. The social consequences that epilepsy can have on people's lives is devastating – people often find that their big problem is not so much the seizures, but how to handle the discrimination and prejudice, which is all too often encountered. Frequently, I would deny my epilepsy at all costs and would not want to talk about it because of society's attitudes.

I went to boarding school when I was 9 years old and it was there that I became very defensive of my epilepsy. I lost the right to take my own medication and I would have to wait in the sick queue along with everyone else to see the matron. I recall the whole school going down with 'flu, and the Deputy Headmaster passing me in the queue saying 'What a long sick list!' 'But Sir,' I shouted back, 'I'm not sick!'

At 16, I was more carefree about my epilepsy, which is very common. I loved beer and rebelled more. I gradually became non-compliant and experienced generalized tonic-clonic seizures for the first time. I knew that the beer drinking coupled with non-compliance would only make my epilepsy worse, but I was in denial and not prepared to take responsibility for myself. My Neanderthal Man theory suggested that people who had epilepsy thousands of years ago (such as Julius Caesar) must have coped without medication and had a life, so why couldn't I?

By the time I was 24, I had been in and out of casualty departments all over the world: from Detroit to Eilat! Until I was 29, I wasn't allowed to drive. On a lighter note, all those years without driving of necessity taught me the quickest way round the underground and how to hitch-hike one's way across Europe fast! The day I passed my test was a memorable one – I had to overcome probably the biggest barrier that someone with epilepsy faces.

In 1988 I joined a support group. Through the group, I began to campaign vigorously to remove the prejudices that people with epilepsy face and spoke at an International Conference in Glasgow in 1992 on 'Attitudes to epilepsy'. There I outlined my belief that it is up to those who have epilepsy to take responsibility for removing the prejudices themselves and not rely upon the work of epilepsy organizations to be solely responsible. The more that people *who already have epilepsy* can acknowledge their epilepsy with friends, the more epilepsy will be better understood. Overall, my experience of living with epilepsy is to accept that one must overcome obstacles to achieve personal ambitions, which would be made easier if I did not have the condition.

From Margaret, a 31-year-old with epilepsy

If I were to choose one phrase to describe my life today, it would most likely be 'I've arrived'. Since my diagnosis at the age of 14 to the present, life has been a battle. With frequent seizures punctuating my life, I always seemed to be engaged in some struggle or other. I went from demanding more independence as a teenager, through struggling against home tuition and then against overprotective tutors at college, and so the list went on . . .

My current feelings of 'Having arrived' have grown out a few events:

- graduating from university with a social work degree;
- being appointed to a permanent post and being able to cope with it;
- having an extremely active social life;
- owning my own home;
- owning a lovely wee car and being legally allowed to drive it.

My survival guide to epilepsy is simple:

- Live according to your own informed choices, not those born of the anxieties of family and friends.
- Set your own personal yardstick for success. Mine was gaining educational fulfilment and being able to hold down a job by doing it well.
- Don't put your life on hold in the hope that things will change. Work around the obstacles so that even the difficult periods of your life will contain an element of achievement.
- Don't feel guilty about making mistakes; just make sure that you learn from them.

From Norman, a 42-year-old man with a family

I was first diagnosed as having epilepsy when I was 7 years old. The slight seizures went away after a short time and it was not until I was 30 that they returned, first as automatisms, then full seizures, both occurring only while I was sleeping.

I remember feeling marked in some way and that I had lost my independence (I could no longer set off round the world, for instance), because I would always need medication and, as this was prescribed monthly, I felt that this was the extent of my freedom.

I know those close to me are affected. The seizures are not pleasant to watch and my wife constantly reminds me to take my medication, even though I do not ever recall forgetting.

I have a very poor short-term memory which can be harrowing, but my greatest fear is that I have passed it on to our daughter who is now 6. There has been no indication yet, but she is so like me when I was a child.

I just keep taking the tablets and only divulge my condition when absolutely necessary.

From Heather, a 40-year-old woman with a family

I would say that there are three basic challenges that epilepsy has presented in my life:

- the unpredictability and effect of my seizures;
- the search for control and management of my condition, and finally
- the legacy of myth and misunderstanding surrounding my epilepsy.

I am frustrated that there is a part of me that is beyond my control, that I have no say in whether I have a simple or complex partial seizure, or whether I have a generalized tonic-clonic seizure. I am a victim of when I have seizures and how long they last. Because I refuse to allow epilepsy to rule my life, I have also made myself a victim of where I have seizures and so must accept the indignity of them in shops, restaurants or at social gatherings. I must also accept the fear of dangers and of seizures when I am alone or in the street. Comments that I heard recently from a 'trained first aider' on being asked what she would do if I had a seizure that I would be dragged my legs, or from another that he would hold me down, do little to inspire me with confidence. The immediate effect of my seizures present their own set of problems for me, such as a disorientation and a loss of awareness of who or where I am, not being able to communicate, physical weakness or overwhelming sickness. This creates an irrational but nonetheless real sense of shame that brings unnecessary tears and apologies.

The challenge of searching for control and management has demanded persistence and fortitude to withstand the horrendous blunders in my early treatment. I have lived through the uncertainty of my epilepsy before it was diagnosed; the pain of surgery and the confusion of the most unlikely diagnoses before my signs and symptoms were recognized for what they really are. Then came the trial and error of drug treatment in the search for a balance in my life which would afford me fewest side effects with the fewest seizures. I still have seizures, I still suffer side effects, but I *am* able to function as near to normal as possible. Living with epilepsy means precisely carrying on within the particular limitations that epilepsy may present – in my case not being permitted to drive or pursue my career – but otherwise, with certain precautions, I carry on as normal.

The legacy of myth and misunderstanding is an aspect of living with epilepsy that is attached to other people and how they see me. Sometimes, their own anxiety and desire to protect are understandable and appreciated, but I have to resist them wrapping me in cottonwool. What is not appreciated is reference to me, or to anyone, as 'an epileptic', as though they reduce my persona to this one feature. Labelling a person like this is anachronistic and associated with the prejudice of previous centuries: that a person with epilepsy is some cursed, pathetic and feeble-minded creature.

Misunderstanding of epilepsy occurs in the medical context as well as in the social context. To be able to live with my epilepsy has meant an education for some medical practitioners as well as for me. My involvement in support and education for people with epilepsy and, in particular, for children and their families and teachers has consistently demonstrated that my own experiences are not unique. Living with epilepsy is a requirement for society and not just the person.

From Jenny, a 35-year-old with epilepsy

I was diagnosed as having epilepsy when I was 18. At the time I was working in a job within the NHS. After 18 months of discussion and union negotiation I was allowed to continue to pursue the work that I enjoyed. Luckily for me, my seizures were controlled by medication and I continued to do all the things that a young adult does and more. As a keen sportswoman I continued to look for leisure pursuits that would test me, pursuits such as hiking, abseiling, canoeing and tall ship sailing.

I started to drive once more. Once I had got my licence back, my social life broadened and life became even more interesting. I started travelling further afield and I was fortunate to tour Australia, ski in Europe and work as a health volunteer for nine weeks in the island communities of Indonesia.

That was 10 years ago; since then a lot has happened and continues to happen. In 1989 I finalized my BSc studies and went off to start another profession. Two years later, I went back to university to continue studying for further qualifications that would enhance my ability to work with children and young people. Now in 1998 I find myself still studying . . .

The career, the leisure pursuits and the qualifications I agree are all desirable and nice to have, but they were hard earned and not without their pitfalls. On reflection, the last 10 years have been exhausting and enjoyable. At times I lost sight of the fact that I had epilepsy and chose to put it on the backburner along with the rest of my health needs. As a consequence, life became a social and academic blur, until finally my body took charge, my seizures became uncontrolled and my general health deteriorated. That happened two years ago, and now at the tender age of 34, I am retired from work and academia owing to ill-health. And no, that does not mean that I am on the social, academic and employment scrapheap, it just means that I am resting and taking stock of my life before I move forward yet again to live my life.

1
What is epilepsy?

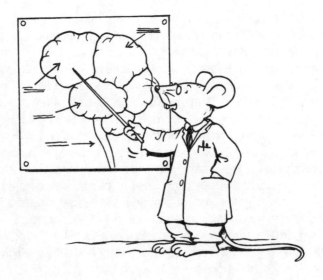

Introduction

When you first hear people talking about epilepsy, you can have the feeling that you are trying to find your way through a maze, with someone speaking in a foreign language as your only guide. Our aim in this chapter is to provide you with a map through the maze, for example by outlining how the brain works, and explaining the many different terms used in epilepsy and how these relate to each other. Obviously everyone is different, and so not every term or example we use in this chapter will relate to you personally. However, you will come across many of them at one time or another, perhaps when talking to other people with epilepsy.

Epilepsy and the brain

What happens in the brains of people who have epilepsy?

To explain this, we need to start by outlining how the brain works. Many people like to think of the brain and how all its nerve cells work as if it was a very complicated computer full of wires and microchips. Others prefer to think of it as a telephone junction box with wires coming in from thousands and thousands of telephones. However, no one could ever build a computer or telephone junction box that was as good as or that could do as much as the human brain.

The brain is made up of thousands of millions of nerve cells called neurons* (we could compare them to the wires in the junction box). Neurons are responsible for controlling all the actions and functions of every part of the body – seeing, hearing, talking, walking and even thinking. As with the computers and junction boxes of our analogy, they work by electricity. Tiny electrical signals are sent along the neurons, between the neurons throughout the brain, and then down into the spinal cord where they can be relayed to any of the other nerves in the body. The links between nerve cells are clearly very important so that they can communicate with each other and pass on the signals.

The actual electrical signals or messages are in the form of chemicals called neurotransmitters ('neuro' means to do with nerve cells and 'transmitters' send or communicate signals or messages). There are many different neurotransmitters within the brain. Some work to cause messages to be sent from one nerve cell to another: these are called excitatory neurotransmitters because they excite or stimulate the neurons. Others work to

---

* There is a glossary at the end of this book to help you with unfamiliar medical terms.

prevent or stop messages being sent: these are called inhibitory neurotransmitters because they inhibit or hold back the signals. Most of the time there is a very close balance between these different types of neurotransmitters.

As with any complicated machine, the brain can sometimes malfunction or develop faults. In epilepsy the fault usually lies in a loss of balance between different neurotransmitters. This can lead to abnormal electrical signals being generated and this electrical activity can progress to a 'seizure'. Seizures take various forms depending upon which areas of the brain are involved. There is more information about seizures in the next two sections of this chapter.

The drugs used to control epilepsy – called antiepileptic or anticonvulsant drugs – work by trying to re-establish the correct balance between the different neurotransmitters.

Does the same part of the brain go wrong in everyone with epilepsy?

No. The brain is organized into different parts, with each part carrying out different functions. The type of epilepsy and the type of seizure depend on what has gone wrong and in which part of the brain.

What do the different parts of the brain do?

The human brain has three major parts: the cerebrum, the cerebellum and the brainstem. They are shown in Figure 1.1.

- *The cerebrum*. This is by far the largest part of the brain and is divided into halves called cerebral hemispheres. The two hemispheres are joined together by the corpus callosum, which is made up of a large number of nerve fibres. The left hemisphere controls everything that happens down the right-hand side of the body, while the right hemisphere controls what happens down the left-hand side. In right-handed people, the left hemisphere is dominant; in left-handed people, the right hemisphere is usually the dominant one. The control of speech and language usually lies within the dominant hemisphere.

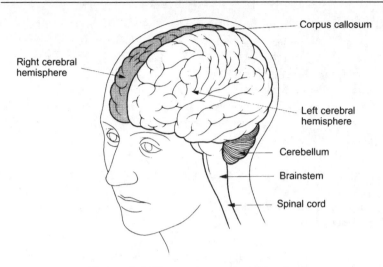

Figure 1.1 The major parts of the brain.

- *The lobes of the cerebrum.* Each of the two cerebral hemi-spheres is divided into four areas: the frontal, parietal, temporal and occipital lobes. They are shown in Figure 1.2. We still have much to learn about precisely what each lobe does, but we do

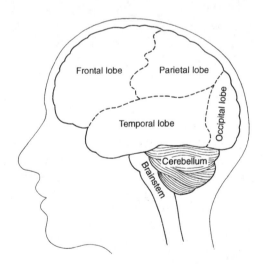

Figure 1.2 The lobes of the cerebrum.

know which lobe is responsible for which of our actions and ways of behaving.

- The frontal lobes are involved in the control of our voluntary movements and some aspects of our behaviour and emotions.
- The parietal lobes are involved in our perception of touch (feeling). They are also involved in skills such as writing and dressing.
- The temporal lobes are involved in memory, speech and language. They are also involved in many aspects of behaviour.
- The occipital lobes are involved in vision and our interpretation of what we see.

- *The cerebellum.* This lies just under the back of the two cerebral hemispheres. It has connections with many other areas of the brain – including the cerebral hemispheres and the brainstem – and with the spinal cord. The cerebellum is involved with the control of movements. These may be large or 'gross' movements (such as walking, jumping and running) or small or 'fine' movements (which include drawing, writing, eating and craftwork). The main function of the cerebellum is to enable all these different movements to take place smoothly and fluently by coordinating the action of all the different muscles. If the cerebellum is damaged or not working properly, then movements become jerky and clumsy (the medical term for this is ataxia) and a tremor may also develop.

- *The brainstem.* This very old and very important part of the brain lies right underneath the cerebral hemispheres. It joins all the other parts of the brain to the spinal cord. It was the first part of the brain to evolve – it existed even in prehistoric times and is found in all primates, i.e. monkeys, apes and humans. Without us being aware of it, it controls breathing and heartbeat, and is involved in the coordination of certain activities including swallowing and eye movements. Without the brainstem we would not be able to live – or do anything!

Types of epilepsy

Is an epileptic seizure the same thing as a fit?

Yes, and you may also hear seizures referred to as convulsions, attacks or turns. People often have their own names for seizures ('wobblers' and a 'funny do' seem to be quite popular ones!). They are all used to describe the same thing – a sudden and uncontrolled episode of excessive electrical activity in the brain. The correct, internationally agreed term for this is seizure, and that is what we have used throughout this book.

Does everyone with epilepsy have the same type of seizure?

No, there are many different types of seizure. The two main types are called generalized seizures and partial seizures.

- *Generalized seizures.* These occur when the abnormal electrical activity that causes a seizure involves both sides of the brain together, as shown in Figure 1.3. Generalized seizures can be further divided into six types. It is important to realize that people with epilepsy may have just one type of generalized seizure or they may have many types:
  - *Absence seizures (or petit mal).* These involve a brief loss of awareness for several (perhaps 5–20) seconds. They usually

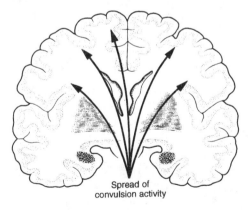

Spread of
convulsion activity

Figure 1.3 Spread of convulsion activity in a generlized seizure.

occur many times a day, every day, and are often accompanied by eyelid fluttering or lip-smacking or chewing movements.

- *Myoclonic seizures.* These involve sudden jerky or shock-like contractions of different muscles anywhere in the body, but usually in the arms or legs. Each myoclonic seizure lasts for a fraction of a second, or for one second at most.
- *Atonic or astatic seizures.* These involve sudden loss of muscle tone, i.e. sudden relaxation of the muscles, resulting in a fall. They often result in a head injury as your head may hit a hard or sharp object such as a desk or table during the fall. An atonic seizure usually lasts for a few seconds, and may be preceded by a very brief myoclonic seizure.
- *Tonic seizures.* These involve sudden stiffness of the limbs or the whole body, again leading to a fall (often like a tree being felled). The seizure usually ends after 5–10 seconds.
- *Clonic seizures.* These involve repeated and rhythmic contractions of the muscles, causing jerks or twitches of the limbs or the whole body. They usually last for between 30 seconds and 1–2 minutes, but sometimes last longer.
- *Tonic-clonic seizures (or grand mal).* These involve a tonic stage followed by a clonic stage, i.e. sudden stiffness and a fall followed by repeated and rhythmic muscle contractions. This pattern of seizure is still commonly called 'grand mal'. Most tonic-clonic seizures last 1–3 minutes; however, some may last for longer, even up to 30 minutes or more (this is then called *status epilepticus*, and is discussed in more detail in Chapter 4).
- *Partial seizures.* These occur when the abnormal electrical activity starts in one lobe of one hemisphere. Figure 1.4 shows how seizures starting in the different lobes can determine the sensations felt. Partial seizures can be further divided into two types called simple and complex.
  - *'Simple'* means that someone's level of consciousness or awareness is not affected during the seizure. Most simple partial seizures involve a change in sensation such as a strange (often unpleasant) smell or taste, or unexplained fear, or a feeling of *déjà vu* (the 'I've been here before' feeling), or even tingling and numbness in the face or an arm. These seizures are called *simple partial sensory seizures.*

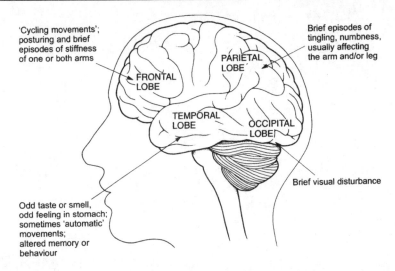

'Cycling movements';
posturing and brief
episodes of stiffness
of one or both arms

PARIETAL
LOBE

FRONTAL
LOBE

Brief episodes of
tingling, numbness,
usually affecting
the arm and/or leg

TEMPORAL
LOBE

OCCIPITAL
LOBE

Brief visual disturbance

Odd taste or smell,
odd feeling in stomach;
sometimes 'automatic'
movements;
altered memory or
behaviour

Figure 1.4 Partial seizures starting in the different lobes determine the sensations felt.

- *'Complex'* means that consciousness or awareness is affected – the person having the seizure may look confused or dazed, or behave or act in a strange way.

If a seizure starts as a partial seizure but then spreads to involve the vast majority of the brain, it is called a *secondary generalized tonic-clonic seizure* (see above), what used to be called 'grand mal' (an example of this is shown in Figure 1.5).

This grouping or classification of the different types of seizure is shown in the diagram in Figure 1.6.

So if there are different types of seizure, does that mean there are different types of epilepsy?

Yes, just as there are different types of seizure, so there are different types of epilepsy, also known as epilepsy syndromes. A syndrome is a cluster of signs and symptoms occurring together in a non-fortuitous, i.e. non-random or non-coincidental, manner. One reason why it is important for doctors to recognize the different types of seizure is that it helps them in turn to recognize different epilepsy syndromes.

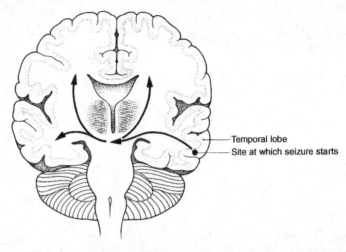

Temporal lobe
Site at which seizure starts

Figure 1.5 The beginning of a partial seizure in the temporal lobe which may then spread (by way of the arrows) to involve the rest of the brain, resulting in a secondary generalized tonic-clonic seizure.

Doctors recognize epilepsy syndromes on the basis of four important pieces of information:

● the type of seizure or seizures experienced;
● the age at which the seizures started – most epilepsy syndromes are age-related, so some are more likely to occur in infancy, some in middle childhood at 5–10 years of age, some in adolescence, and some in adult life;

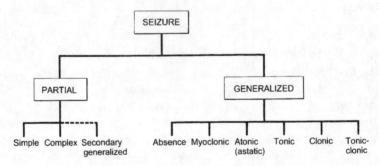

Figure 1.6 Seizure classification.

- the person's development or learning abilities; and
- what the electroencephalograph (EEG) shows (see *EEGs* in Chapter 2).

It is only when all of these pieces of information are studied that an epilepsy syndrome can be recognized or identified. However, only about 50–65% of people will be found to have a clear-cut epilepsy syndrome.

Another way of grouping epilepsy is by how much, if anything is known about what caused it. Here there are three different groups:

- In *idiopathic* or *primary epilepsy* no obvious cause can be found. We suspect that many idiopathic epilepsies may eventually be found to have a genetic basis (see *Possible causes* later in this chapter).
- In *cryptogenic epilepsy* a cause is suspected but none can actually be found!
- In *symptomatic* or *secondary epilepsy* there is a known cause. For example, the epilepsy may have started after an infection involving the brain, e.g. meningitis or encephalitis, or after a head injury, or because the brain has never developed properly.

I don't see how all these different classifications fit together. Can you please explain?

Doctors can combine terms from the different classifications to describe a particular type of epilepsy. The description will often include terms describing the cause of the epilepsy, the type of seizure involved and the age when it started. For example, the description 'idiopathic generalized tonic-clonic epilepsy' tells us that the cause is not known (idiopathic), that the seizures affect both sides of the brain (generalized) and that they involve sudden stiffness and a fall followed by repeated rhythmic muscle contractions (tonic-clonic). Similarly the term 'juvenile myoclonic epilepsy' tells us that the epilepsy came on in late childhood or adolescence (the juvenile time of life!) and that the seizures include jerky muscle contractions (myoclonic).

There are internationally agreed standards for these descriptions, and by following them doctors can ensure that they all know exactly which type of epilepsy is being discussed. Obviously some descriptions will be more common than others, as some types of epilepsy and epilepsy syndromes are more common than others.

Just to make things more complicated, one or two epilepsy syndromes (usually the rarer ones) are known not by these classification descriptions but are instead named after the doctors who first studied them! One example is West syndrome, named after a Dr West. This syndrome is discussed in a later question.

This all strikes me as horribly complicated and I can't see why all these groupings are needed. Why can't we just call it epilepsy and get on with treating it?

You are not alone in finding it complicated – even some doctors find it a little confusing, particularly those who are not experienced in treating epilepsy. But it is important to try and recognize, i.e. classify, the specific type of epileptic seizure and the specific epilepsy or epilepsy syndrome, for two main reasons. When an epilepsy syndrome cannot be identified, then the type of epilepsy is usually classified on the type of seizure.

The first reason is to give us information on your prognosis, i.e. on the outlook or expected outcome. You and your doctors need to know whether the seizures will be easily controlled with medication and if there is the possibility that the seizures and the epilepsy may eventually 'go away'. Some types of seizure and some epilepsy syndromes have a better prognosis than others.

The second reason is that knowing which type of epilepsy it is will help guide the doctors in choosing the most appropriate antiepileptic drug to treat you. For example, some drugs appear to be more effective in treating partial seizures whilst others are better at treating generalized seizures.

My GP doesn't use any of the terms you use, he says I have petit mal. Does this mean I don't actually have epilepsy?

No, it means that your doctor is using an older term for what is now called *absence epilepsy*. Unfortunately, many people (doctors included) use the term 'petit mal' for both absence and complex partial seizures. The terms used to describe epilepsy have changed over the years and, although the newer terms are more accurate, some people still use the older terms out of habit, or because they sound less technical, or because they are easier to remember. Table 1.1 gives the modern equivalents for some of the more commonly used older terms. You will find descriptions of all these types of seizures under their current names earlier in this section.

Table 1.1 Modern terms for some older epilepsy terms

Old name	Current name
petit mal	absence
jerk	myoclonic
drop	atonic or astatic
stiffening	tonic
repeated jerking	clonic
grand mal	tonic-clonic

What is the Lennox–Gastaut syndrome?

This is a specific and rare type of epilepsy syndrome which starts in childhood. The outlook is not good. Children may need special schooling or, rarely, care in a residential centre for people with severe epilepsy.

It is named after the two eminent experts in epilepsy who first described it. As with any epilepsy syndrome, it has a number of features which help doctors to identify it:

● The age at which the seizures start, which is usually between the ages of 2 and 6 years old, but it can occasionally start in children who are 1–2 years old, or in those aged around 7 or 8.

● The types of seizures, usually of several kinds, including tonic, atonic, tonic-clonic, myoclonic and secondary generalized tonic-clonic seizures (see above). There may be atypical absence seizures – where people appear confused, unresponsive, not talking and perhaps wandering around doing strange things for many minutes – very different from typical absence seizures during which awareness is simply lost for a number of seconds.

● The EEG shows a characteristic pattern (called slow spike and slow wave activity) which usually occurs over the whole brain and not just one part of it. EEGs are discussed in more detail in Chapter 2.

There are many different causes of Lennox–Gastaut syndrome, for example an abnormal development of the brain before birth or following on from meningitis as a baby, or brain damage occurring around the time of birth.

Some children with this syndrome will have had another rare type of epilepsy called infantile spasms or West syndrome in their first year of life and will then go on to have the Lennox–Gastaut syndrome before their second or third birthday. However, a definite cause will only be found in about 50–60% of people with the syndrome.

Unfortunately Lennox–Gastaut syndrome is a severe form of epilepsy. The seizures are very difficult to control and very few children ever have all the different seizure types fully controlled for more than a few weeks or months at a time. Because of this, most of the antiepileptic drugs are tried, often in combination with each other. If there are very frequent atonic or tonic-clonic seizures (often occurring many times a day), then a surgical procedure called a corpus callosotomy may occasionally be considered. This involves division of the corpus callosum, the part of the brain which joins together the two cerebral hemispheres, and it may in some people result in stopping these types of seizures or at least reducing their frequency.

Learning and behaviour will also be affected. Almost 90% of children who have Lennox–Gastaut syndrome will already have had development problems or learning difficulties when the seizures start. After one, two or three years of having seizures, all children with the syndrome have learning and behaviour difficulties – often severe. This usually happens even if the child's seizures are quite well-controlled. These difficulties usually continue into adulthood and throughout the person's life.

More about seizures

My father who is 70 has just developed epilepsy. I thought only children developed epilepsy?

As people get older it has been realized that small strokes and other illnesses can make somebody more likely to have seizures – the highest incidence of epilepsy now is in old age. Nevertheless, seizures developing in older people do tend to be easier to treat and we would normally use the same drugs as in younger people.

Can you have a seizure without having epilepsy?

Yes, and many people will have at least one seizure during their lives. Doctors will only diagnose epilepsy if seizures have been unprovoked and have occurred two or three times. The diagnosis of epilepsy is discussed in Chapter 2.

Can people get warnings of seizures?

Yes, when epilepsy starts from any of the lobes of the brain, particularly the temporal lobe, people often experience a warning that a seizure is about to happen. (The lobes of the brain are shown in Figure 1.2 earlier in this chapter.) This warning usually involves a strange sensation, feeling, smell or taste and is known as an 'aura'. An aura is actually a simple partial sensory seizure. The most common warning sensations are:

- *paraesthesia* (pins and needles) in one or more limbs, which may spread up the limb, e.g. from the toes to the hip, or from the fingers to the shoulder and face;
- *epigastric sensations* (unpleasant feelings or sensations in the stomach);
- *gustatory-olfactory sensations* (strange tastes or smells);
- *fear* or *panic*;
- a feeling of *déjà vu* (the 'I've been here before' feeling);
- *visual or auditory hallucinations* (seeing or hearing strange things).

Is there anything that can trigger a seizure?

Failing to take antiepileptic drugs regularly, becoming overtired, and having too much alcohol, too little sleep or a high temperature or fever are all examples of situations where a seizure may be more likely to happen. In that sense we could say that these examples could be considered 'triggers' for epilepsy.

However, there is also a rare group of epilepsies called *reflex epilepsies* in which a seizure can occur in response to a specific trigger or stimulus. The best-known of these (because it has received so much media publicity in the last few years) is photosensitivity, and this is discussed in the answer to the next question. Very few people have reflex epilepsy; even if they do, they rarely encounter any of the triggering factors.

I remember seeing a lot of reports on the television about the flashing patterns in computer games bringing on epilepsy. Will these affect me?

Only if you are photosensitive. Photosensitivity means being sensitive or susceptible to flashing or flickering lights, but only when the flashes or flickers occur at a certain frequency. It may occur in isolation but is far more commonly seen in people with epilepsy – usually idiopathic (also called primary) generalized epilepsy. Photosensitivity usually develops at between 6 and 18 years of age, with a peak at 12–16 years old; it tends to affect girls more often than boys and is now realized to be lifelong.

Seizures can be triggered in those with photosensitive epilepsy by:

- flashing lights (often with 12–20 flashes per second);
- strobe lighting (often found in discos or amusement arcades);
- sunlight shining through a row of trees, railings or buildings as the person passes by in a car or bus or, occasionally, if the person is running fast past them;
- strongly striped or geometric patterns.

It is important to realize that flashing lights, television sets and computer games do *not* make a person photosensitive or cause epilepsy. They are only able to trigger or provoke a seizure in someone who is already susceptible, or who already has epilepsy. In fact, only about 4–5% of *all* people with epilepsy are photosensitive.

Doctors can find out whether or not you are photosensitive by performing an EEG (see **EEGs** in Chapter 2). If you are, then there are practical ways of handling the problem in Chapter 9.

We are often told that we lead more stressful lives these days. How does this affect people with epilepsy – will it make them have more seizures?

Stress in itself rarely provokes a seizure. However, if you are in a stressful situation (e.g. worrying about your job or family problems), then this may well have an adverse effect on sleeping patterns and general health, which in turn may lower your seizure threshold and make a seizure more likely to happen.

We all need to develop ways of handling stress, whether or not we have epilepsy – it is a natural part of life and it is impossible for any of us to avoid it completely. Your worry that stress will provoke seizures is very natural, but it will not actually do you very much good. It would be better to talk about your worries and decide how you can best cope with them. You can also help by looking after your general health, for example by making sure that you eat a healthy diet and take regular exercise.

My epilepsy is much worse around my periods. Is there a reason for this?

Some women and girls complain that their seizures are worse at the start of or just before their periods. Seizures which are caused or made worse by menstruation (periods) are called *catamenial seizures*. Your specialist may be able to adjust your antiepileptic drugs to allow for these catamenial seizures.

It is possible that cyclical changes in seizure frequency may well be related to specific times in the monthly menstrual cycle. One suggested cause is the rapid fall in levels of progesterone (one of the female sex hormones) which naturally occurs at or immediately before a period.

Can people have epilepsy in their sleep?

Yes, people can have seizures during sleep. Some only ever have seizures when they are asleep at night and never during the day when they are awake. Some types of epilepsy are commonly associated with seizures that occur during sleep (complex partial seizures, particularly if they arise from the frontal lobes) or just after waking (juvenile myoclonic epilepsy, JME).

Because most people sleep at night, these seizures are described as *nocturnal seizures*, although they can occur whenever someone is asleep. We do not yet know the reason for them, but we do know that, when the brain is relatively inactive (as during some parts of sleep), then it is more likely that a seizure will occur. This is why EEG tests are sometimes done during sleep or after a period of sleep deprivation – it increases the chance of abnormal electrical signals showing up (see **EEGs** in Chapter 2).

I have occasionally wet myself when I have a seizure. Why?

It is difficult to give you a precise reason without knowing what type of seizure you have, but we can give you a general answer. You can have such accidents, called *urinary incontinence*, during two types of seizure. The first and more common of these is a generalized tonic-clonic seizure, because during this type of seizure there can be a sudden and often disordered contraction of the abdominal and bladder muscles. If these contractions are very disordered there can even be some faecal incontinence, i.e. when you can dirty or soil yourself.

The other type of seizure in which urinary incontinence can occur is a complex partial seizure, although this is uncommon. In this type of seizure you are not fully aware of where you are or what you are doing, and so you may try and urinate (pass water) inappropriately, i.e. in the wrong place and at the wrong time.

I was talking to someone in the hospital waiting room, and her seizures sounded different from my own. But we'd both been told that the seizures are complex partial ones, so why the differences?

Our explanation has to be very general, because we don't know enough about either of your seizures to be more specific. You have been told that you have complex partial seizures – 'complex' meaning that there is some loss of or alteration in consciousness (awareness) during a seizure, and 'partial' meaning that the seizures start in only one part of the brain. The differences that you and the other person have noticed suggest that, although you both have complex partial seizures, these seizures may be starting in different places in the brain. Exactly where in the brain a seizure starts will determine what happens during it.

Complex partial seizures can occasionally start in one or other of the frontal lobes (the different lobes are shown in Figure 1.2). However, they *usually* start in the temporal lobes, which is why you may sometimes hear the description 'temporal lobe epilepsy'. The temporal lobes control particularly emotion, memory, speech and language: exactly what happens during a complex partial seizure will depend upon which part of the temporal lobe is involved. The seizures may be associated with unexpected movements, strange feelings, fluctuating emotions or altered behaviour. As well as this, complex partial seizures may spread to involve the whole brain, when they are known as secondary generalized tonic-clonic seizures and have different effects again.

My brother is the only person I know with epilepsy. When he has a seizure he goes unconscious, falls down and then shakes all over. Is this typical – do all people with epilepsy do this?

As you can see from other answers in this chapter, there are many different types of seizure, so the answer to the second part of your question is no, not all people have the type of seizure you describe.

To answer the first part of your question, your brother's seizures are typical of a particular type of epilepsy called generalized tonic-clonic seizures. During this type of seizure the body will stiffen; there may be a cry or grunt (not of pain), followed by a fall, and then the convulsion begins. Your brother may go blue (cyanosed) because of lack of oxygen, he may drool or froth at the mouth (also called salivation), he may wet himself, and there will be rhythmic jerking movements of all his limbs – this is the shaking you describe.

This type of seizure usually lasts between one and three minutes and usually stops by itself. Occasionally, in very severe cases, drugs such as diazepam (brand names for this drug include Valium, Diazepam Rectubes and Stesolid) may have to be given to stop the seizure. See also *Antiepileptic drugs* in Chapter 3 and *First aid* in Chapter 4.

Why does he turn blue during a seizure?

Not everyone turns blue during a generalized tonic-clonic seizure, but it can occasionally happen. When it occurs, it is usually most noticeable around the lips and mouth – it is then called perioral cyanosis.

The blueness is due to the fact that during the seizure the breathing becomes irregular and, because of this, not enough oxygen fills his lungs. When this happens the blood going to all his tissues and organs (including the skin, which is an organ) is not quite as pink as it usually is, and therefore the skin can turn a little blue. Usually it only takes two or three minutes for breathing to become more regular, and then the oxygen within the lungs and within the blood rapidly becomes normal and the skin quickly turns pink again.

Are there any risks of long-term damage to health from having seizures?

This is a difficult question to answer as so many factors have to be taken into consideration, including the type of epilepsy, what is known about its cause, and whether there are any other medical problems as well as epilepsy. At one end of the scale there are those who have seizures only occasionally, and of a type which usually 'go away' as they grow up: for them, we can say that there are few or no risks of any long-term health damage. At the other end of the scale are those with severe epilepsy and other major problems, and for them we can only say that the risks are much greater. In general, the effects of epilepsy on a person's long-term health will be less favourable in the following circumstances:

- if the epilepsy began at under 2 years old;
- if the cause of the epilepsy is known, e.g. brain damage from a head injury;
- if there are associated neurological abnormalities or disorders, i.e. other problems affecting the brain or nervous system, such as learning difficulties or cerebral palsy;

- if the type of seizure includes myoclonic, tonic or atonic seizures;
- if initial seizure control was difficult;
- if more than one antiepileptic drug is needed to control the seizures;
- if episodes of convulsive status epilepticus have occurred (see Chapter 4 for more information about status epilepticus).

Rarely, someone can die in a seizure. It tends to be people with severe frequent tonic-clonic seizures who may be found dead in bed. The fatal seizure is usually not witnessed.

Possible causes

Do we know what causes epilepsy?

In about 50% of cases diagnosed as having epilepsy, no specific cause for it will be found. This is why so many types of epilepsy are described as being 'idiopathic', which simply means that the cause is not known. It seems likely that some of these idiopathic forms of epilepsy may have a genetic cause, and this is discussed in the answer to the next question.

Epilepsy can be due to virtually anything which affects the brain, and seizures may also occur in association with many other disorders which do not affect the brain directly. For example, epilepsy may start after an infection involving the brain, e.g. meningitis or encephalitis, or after a head injury, or because the brain has never developed properly, or because of cerebral hypoxia (lack of oxygen to a baby's brain) at birth. When a cause is known, the epilepsy is described as being 'symptomatic' or 'secondary'.

Can you inherit epilepsy?

A lot of research is going on at the moment into the links between different medical conditions, not just epilepsy, and our genetic makeup (the characteristics we inherit from our parents). More and more conditions are turning out to have a genetic cause, and epilepsy is probably no different. There are many different types of epilepsy, and some of these types of epilepsy may have a genetic basis.

Genes are the parts of a human cell which determine which characteristics you inherit from your parents. In other words, the cells in your body contain sets of instructions (genes) which control the ways in which the cells grow and behave.

Things can go wrong with these sets of instructions (they are then called abnormal genes), and it may be that one or more abnormal genes are responsible for causing epilepsy. If a child happens to inherit one or more of these abnormal genes from the parents, then the child may develop epilepsy. The particular genes a child gets from each parent are a matter of chance, and this applies just as much to abnormal genes as to the ones which determine the colour of our eyes or the size of our feet.

It is also important to realize that one or both parents may simply be carrying one of the abnormal genes without necessarily having epilepsy themselves. In this situation, epilepsy may still develop in their child or children.

We do know that inheritance plays a part in one particular type of epilepsy called *primary generalized epilepsy*. If someone in the family (a parent or a brother or sister) has this type of epilepsy, then the chances of another child in the family having a similar type of epilepsy are increased ten-fold. If there is no family history of this type of epilepsy, then a child has at most a 0.5–1% chance of developing it, i.e. approximately one child in every 100–200 children. Other types of epilepsy and other epilepsy syndromes carry different and often much lower risks of inheritance.

Can other conditions that affect the brain cause epilepsy?

Epilepsy is far more common in those who have other conditions which affect the brain. These conditions include cerebral palsy, learning difficulties, cerebrovascular disease (stroke) and dementia. All of these conditions have different causes, but the common link between them is a brain abnormality, i.e. something has gone wrong in the brain or the brain has been damaged in some way. It is the brain abnormality, whatever its cause, which is responsible for causing all these problems, including any epilepsy. However, none of these conditions actually *causes* epilepsy, and neither does epilepsy cause cerebral palsy, learning difficulties, behaviour problems and so on.

Unfortunately, the epilepsy which occurs in association with any of these other medical conditions is likely to be more severe and more difficult to control with antiepileptic drugs. Conditions which are usually linked to difficult epilepsy include cerebral palsy, tuberous sclerosis and severe learning difficulties. Infections which affect the brain, e.g. meningitis or encephalitis, may also lead to difficult epilepsy.

Epilepsy may also be caused by a head injury, although this is rare. It usually follows only a bad or serious head injury that led to a long period of unconsciousness or loss of memory; or one in which the skull was fractured and the edge of the broken skull bone was forced downwards into the brain; or one that caused a blood clot to develop in the brain.

Brain tumours cause epilepsy in about six out of every 100 cases, but this figure is lower in children, with only one or two cases per 100.

There is an increased incidence of epilepsy in the elderly, particularly those who have cerebrovascular disease or dementia (about 10%).

Facts and figures

How many people have epilepsy?

In this country, approximately 350 000–400 000 people of all ages currently have epilepsy; of these some 90 000–100 000 are children aged anywhere from a few months old to 16 years old. As the proportion of a population with a particular medical condition at any one time is referred to as the 'prevalence', we could say that the prevalence of epilepsy among people in this country is 0.5–0.8%.

The 'incidence' of a condition is the number of people developing it for the first time during each year, i.e. the number of new cases within a year. The incidence of epilepsy varies, depending upon the age of the person. It is highest in the first year of life: in any one year approximately 140 children in every 100 000 who are under a year old will be diagnosed with epilepsy. This figure falls to 40 people in every 100 000 in adult life. In the elderly, the incidence rises to 150 in 100 000 in those aged 70–79 years.

Is there more epilepsy around these days? If so, is there anything we can do to prevent it?

Epilepsy does not appear to be on the increase except amongst the elderly, as people live longer. A small proportion of epilepsy is preventable, e.g. by taking sensible safety measures to protect people from severe head injuries or by treating quickly any infections which may affect the brain, e.g. meningitis or ence-phalitis. However, as we do not know the cause of most epilepsies (although we suspect it may have a genetic basis – see above), it is largely unpreventable.

Is epilepsy more common in women than in men, or vice versa?

When you look at all types of epilepsy at all ages, there is no major difference between males and females in terms of the incidence or prevalence of epilepsy. However, there are certain types of epilepsy which are more common in females than in males, for example absence epilepsy. Photosensitivity is also more common in females.

Is it true that epilepsy is linked to high intelligence?

No. It is important to realize that epilepsy can occur in anyone with below average, average or above average intelligence. However, those who had brain damage or in whom the brain never developed properly, and those who have learning difficulties or cerebral palsy, or both, are much more likely to have a severe form of epilepsy and also to have seizures which may persist for most of their lives.

2
Diagnosing epilepsy

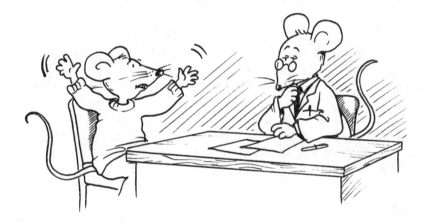

Introduction

It is obviously crucial to establish a correct diagnosis of epilepsy, as without this it will be impossible for your doctor to plan which investigations need to be done, decide which treatment will be most suitable, or predict what might happen in the future. The diagnosis of epilepsy may be either easy or difficult to make. It is

There is a glossary at the end of this book to help you with unfamiliar medical terms.

33

usually made on taking a good description of the 'event', particularly from people who saw what happened. There is no one test which will absolutely confirm or deny epilepsy, so doctors have to take many factors into account. This can mean that the process of diagnosis can sometimes seem long and frustrating. Understanding what is going on can help to make the process feel less tedious, and we hope that the explanations in this chapter will help with this.

How do they know that it's epilepsy?

What tests are needed to diagnose epilepsy?

The diagnosis of epilepsy is always a clinical diagnosis, i.e. it is mainly based on what the doctor is told and on the information that you can provide – you, and perhaps your partner, will be asked a great many questions! EEGs (a special test recording brain waves) can provide useful additional information, particularly about the type of epilepsy or epilepsy syndrome; some people also need brain scans. There are separate sections on *EEGs* and *Scans* later in this chapter; in this section we concentrate on the information the doctors need to make a clinical diagnosis of epilepsy.

Making a correct clinical diagnosis of epilepsy can take some time, and it is very unlikely that any harm will come to you by waiting. It is very important that the diagnosis is correct, as a wrong diagnosis can lead to future problems. Should a seizure occur, then your GP will probably refer you to a specialist at your local hospital. Most cases will be seen at the hospital within four to six weeks, and some are seen earlier than this.

My sister told me what had happened when I first had a seizure. Should she come along as well when I visit the doctor?

Yes, she should. Before a diagnosis can be made, a doctor needs to be given a very clear, detailed and accurate account of precisely what happened during a seizure. It is therefore essential that the person who has actually seen the seizure (the eyewitness) should go along to give the doctor this very important information. In your case, the eyewitness is your sister.

Your doctor will have to ask many questions about what actually happened before, during and after your seizure. The sequence of events should be described as accurately as possible. If this information (called the history) is unclear or incomplete, then a diagnosis of epilepsy must not be made and the doctor must wait for more information.

The most common reason for a mistaken or wrong diagnosis of epilepsy is that someone has failed to take a detailed and accurate history of what happened to someone during a seizure and has then jumped to the wrong conclusion. Usually this is because no one can remember what happened just before the seizure began.

Your sister should not worry if she is unable to remember every detail of what happened to you – she would be an exceptional person if she could!. She should simply do her best to answer your doctor's questions as fully as possible. No harm will come to you if you have to wait a while for a diagnosis, and your doctor will have been alerted to your condition.

All I can remember about my sister's first seizure is being in a complete state of panic, I was so frightened. I managed to call the doctor, but I simply wasn't able to describe properly what had happened. Did I do the right thing?

Yes, you did. It is not surprising that in the circumstances you were unable to remember every detail of what happened to your sister, and the way you felt was not unusual.

A number of research studies have clearly shown that, when people first see a tonic-clonic seizure, they actually think that the person is going to die, and they feel utterly helpless. This common response indicates the degree of anxiety felt by anyone when a seizure is witnessed. It is important to realize that it is rare for anyone to die during a seizure.

When someone has a seizure for the first time, contact the GP as soon as possible. In the vast majority the seizure will have stopped by the time that the doctor gets there. If for some reason the GP is not available, then it is entirely reasonable to call an ambulance and have the person taken to the Accident and Emergency department of the nearest hospital. If a seizure lasts for more than 10–15 minutes then this is an emergency and an ambulance must be called immediately. There is more about emergencies in Chapter 4.

How does anyone ever remember enough details about a seizure to be able to describe it to a doctor?

It is very common for eyewitnesses not to be able to remember exactly what happened when someone had a seizure. Eye-witnesses seeing a seizure for the first time may be under-standably frightened and may actually think that the person is going to die, and because of this they cannot remember the exact sequence of events.

By the time the specialist is seen at a hospital, it may have been some days or even weeks since the seizure and the eyewitnesses may have forgotten what actually happened. Doctors are well used to this happening, and will usually ask questions to jog the eyewitnesses' memories and help them remember as many details as possible.

If you can overcome your initial panic, then, if you see another seizure, it would be useful for you to write down as soon as you can all the details of what happened in the exact order in which they occurred – use of a seizure diary as mentioned later may help.

Another very useful way of providing an accurate description of a seizure is to get someone to film or record one with a camcorder, if you have one. The specialist would find such a video extremely useful, to help not only in making a correct diagnosis of epilepsy but also in establishing the specific type of seizure and epilepsy.

Miming or acting out how someone moved or behaved during a seizure can also help, as it is often easier to show a doctor what happened than to try to describe it in words. The doctor may even do the miming for you!

Our family doctor is very good at discussing things with us and she always explains exactly what is going on. When she was told about my first seizure, she said she was not sure whether or not it was epilepsy, although it might be, so she is referring me to a specialist at the hospital. Why doesn't she know for sure – is it very difficult for doctors to diagnose epilepsy?

Yes, it can be. The first problem is that there are a number of other conditions which can produce episodes or attacks which may resemble or look like an epileptic seizure. These are discussed in the answer to the next question. It is obviously very important for a doctor to know that these conditions exist and what may happen when a seizure occurs. However, as family doctors have to know a lot about many different conditions, it is not surprising that many GPs do not know about these specific ones in detail, in particular the similarities and differences between the attacks caused by them and the attacks caused by epilepsy.

Another reason why it may be difficult to make a precise diagnosis is that there are many different types of epileptic seizure, and many different types of epilepsy and epilepsy syndromes. Some seizures are very obvious and are easily recognized, e.g. a generalized tonic-clonic seizure or an atonic seizure. All the different types of seizure mentioned here are discussed in more detail in Chapter 1. Other seizures may be more subtle and therefore more difficult to recognize, e.g. a brief absence seizure, where someone may just appear to stare into space for some seconds, a brief myoclonic seizure, which may be simply a sudden or momentary jerk of the head or body, or a complex partial seizure, which may just show itself by the person appearing a little confused and behaving rather strangely.

As we have explained in the earlier answers in this section, the information that is most needed in making a diagnosis of epilepsy is a precise description of what happened during a seizure, and eyewitnesses cannot always remember the exact details. When you take all these factors into account, it is not surprising that your GP was a little unsure about making a firm diagnosis. She therefore did the sensible thing and referred you for a second opinion – *all* people with suspected epilepsy should be seen by a specialist.

The specialist whom you will see may be a neurologist (one who specializes in the brain and nervous system) or a general physician, if a neurologist is not available. Whatever the label, the specialist will have a wider understanding and knowledge of the different sorts of epilepsy than your GP, and should be able to decide whether you have epilepsy or some other non-epileptic condition. Clearly, this sounds far quicker and easier than it will be in real life! The diagnosis of epilepsy is never a snap judgement. Instead, as you would expect, the specialist will need to ask a lot of questions and perhaps carry out some tests before making a definite diagnosis.

What other conditions can be mistaken for epilepsy?

Fainting, migraine, hyperventilation and pseudoseizures (also called pseudo-epileptic seizures or non-epileptic attacks) are the most common causes of misdiagnosis.

- *Benign paroxysmal vertigo.* People may mention that the room appears to be spinning around. After a number of seconds this feeling and any fear goes away and normality quickly returns. People are not confused or sleepy after these attacks.
- *Simple faints.* Also called syncopal or vasovagal attacks, these are very common, particularly in teenage girls. Faints usually occur if someone has been standing in a hot room for a long time, or is unwell with a bad cold or stomach upset. They feel dizzy, sweaty, unwell and perhaps sick, and friends comment that they look 'deathly white' before they fall. There may be some very brief jerky movements when they are on the floor. Very rarely there may be urinary incontinence, i.e. people may wet themselves. Recovery is usually very quick, within a few minutes. Faints are due to a very slow heart rate, and the heart rate always speeds up when someone is lying down.
- *Migraine.* This severe type of headache is sometimes preceded by a visual aura. Although auras may also occur in epilepsy, the aura before a migraine headache lasts for longer than an epileptic aura (see *More about seizures* in Chapter 1).

- *Narcolepsy.* Episodes of suddenly falling asleep anywhere and anytime for anything between 30 seconds and a few minutes.
- *Paroxysmal choreoathetosis.* A group of very rare conditions provoked by emotional stress or sudden movement, during which people show rather strange writhing and twisting movements of the limbs.
- *Cardiac dysrhythmias.* Abnormalities of heart rate or rhythm.
- *Hyperventilation.* Overbreathing, i.e. breathing too hard or too fast, often because of a panic attack.
- *Pseudoseizures.* Also called pseudo-epileptic seizures or non-epileptic attacks, these are seizures which look like epileptic seizures but are not. They often have an underlying psychological cause, and are much more common in females than in males.

I went to the hospital recently with my girlfriend and the doctor said that some of her seizures might not be epilepsy. She mentioned something called pseudoseizures. What are these?

These are seizures that look like epilepsy, but normally have a psychological cause. They are called many things, but doctors often now prefer the term non-epileptic attacks.

We now know that they are more common than once thought. Some people only have non-epileptic attacks, but others like your girlfriend have both non- and true epileptic seizures. When there is a mix like this, it can be especially difficult to tell the difference between each type.

It is often difficult too to find out why people have non-epileptic attacks, but the reasons must be pursued so that a relevant treatment programme can be started. Antiepileptic drugs will not work but, where there are true epileptic seizures also, the drug(s) should be continued for these.

Preferably, treatment should not be decided upon until a person has been assessed by a neuropsychologist; however, one or more of the following may be tried dependent on the cause:

- ignoring and avoiding rewarding attacks;
- positive reinforcement for attack-free periods;

- behavioural management;
- anger management;
- environmental manipulation, and
- counselling.

Treatment can be successful, but it may take a lengthy period and it is true to say some doctors are not keen to manage non-epileptic attacks.

The specialist at the hospital asked exactly the same questions as our GP – why the duplication?

Because obtaining as much information as possible about what actually happened is of such great importance in the diagnosis of epilepsy or in the diagnosis of those other conditions which may, at first glance, appear to be epilepsy. We realize that it can be very frustrating to go over the same thing again and again, but it cannot be stressed enough just how important this information is. It is usual to think that we have remembered everything, but it can help to go over events more than once, as sometimes it helps us to remember some small detail which may seem insignificant to us but which may be very significant to the doctor. It is crucial to get the facts right and that is why different doctors will often ask exactly the same questions!

Apparently, there were a lot of questions about my health when I was a baby. How can what happened so many years ago be relevant to making a diagnosis now?

The doctor needs a complete picture of your present state of health and to get this it is often necessary to go back, even as far as your birth, in order to find out as much information as possible. This enables the doctor to put together all the pieces of the 'diagnostic jigsaw' and so make the correct diagnosis. For example, you may have had a head injury in the past, or an illness which can affect the brain, e.g. meningitis and encephalitis, and these could be relevant to your present condition. Epilepsy can also be a symptom of many different underlying disorders, and knowing as much as possible about your medical history will help the doctor rule these out or decide if further tests are needed.

Apart from answering all those questions you've mentioned, what else can we expect when I go to see the specialist?

The specialist will probably want to give you a careful physical examination, and take some blood for testing. All these tests will provide information about your current state of health and help the specialist reach a correct diagnosis.

These tests and examinations are important, although they are rarely helpful in deciding whether or not seizures are actually due to epilepsy – most people with epilepsy have normal test results – but they can help in finding if there is an underlying cause. Seizures may be a symptom of another problem, such as a low blood level of glucose or calcium, and this would show up in a blood test. Tests can also help in identifying a particular epilepsy syndrome, when information about previous development is needed as well as information about the seizure type, or in establishing whether or not you have another medical condition as well as epilepsy.

You may also have an EEG and a brain scan; there are sections on both these tests later in this chapter.

I do not think that my epilepsy diagnosis is correct. What should I do? Is it possible to get a second opinion?

You do not say whether the diagnosis was made by your GP or by a specialist. If it was your GP, then you could ask for referral to a specialist at your local hospital (in our opinion, *everyone* with suspected epilepsy should be seen by a specialist). If you are already under the care of a hospital specialist, then in the first instance you should talk over your concerns about the diagnosis with him or her. If after this discussion you are still unhappy, then it is reasonable for you to ask for another opinion.

These suggestions are based on the assumption that you simply want to make sure that the diagnosis is correct. What we cannot tell from your question is whether you are instead asking for help in coming to terms with the diagnosis. Being told that you have epilepsy is a shock, and disbelief is a common reaction. If this is the case, then we would still suggest that talking things through with your specialist would be a good starting point. A few specialists work with trained counsellors and many have epilepsy nurse specialists who can listen to your worries and concerns (see also *Coming to terms with epilepsy* in Chapter 5; you may find this section helpful).

EEGs

What exactly is an EEG?

An EEG (encephalogram) is a test which records and measures the tiny electrical signals (sometimes called 'brainwaves') produced inside the brain. It provides a picture of the electrical activity inside the brain, whether it be the normal activity that goes on all the time or the 'out of the correct order' activity that occurs during a seizure (see *Epilepsy and the brain* in Chapter 1).

During an EEG, small discs called electrodes are placed on the head. Usually 32 electrodes are required. These electrodes pick up the brainwaves and transfer them to the EEG machine where they are amplified (enlarged). They are then displayed on a TV screen or recorded on paper or computer disk.

The EEG recording consists of several lines, and each line is a picture of the brainwaves being produced by a different part of the brain (determined by the placing of the electrodes). This means that the EEG can show not only what is happening, but also where in the brain it is happening.

An EEG is completely painless. The electricity goes only from the brain to the machine, not the other way around, so there is absolutely no risk of getting an electric shock. A routine EEG in the out-patient department of a hospital takes from 30–90 minutes to complete. The main complaint about EEGs is the hairwashing that is needed afterwards – the electrodes sometimes have to be stuck to the head with a special glue! However, it is possible for the electrodes to be held in place by other techniques, including something that looks like a rubber hairnet.

What part do EEGs play in making a diagnosis of epilepsy?

They are invaluable tools in the investigation and classification of epilepsy, provided that they are recorded carefully and interpreted correctly. They are *not* a substitute for a clinical diagnosis, i.e. one based on what the doctor observes and on the information that you or an eyewitness provide. EEGs should never be interpreted in isolation but always in conjunction with what is happening clinically. In other words, they should only be used to support a clinical diagnosis of epilepsy, and to help decide what type of seizure is involved. Doctors combine the information provided by EEGs with what is known about a seizure type or types to help them find out if you have a particular type of epilepsy or epilepsy syndrome (see *Types of epilepsy* in Chapter 1).

If EEGs are so useful, why shouldn't they be used on their own to confirm an epilepsy diagnosis?

Because they have their limitations as well as their uses. As almost 50% of people with epilepsy have normal EEGs between seizures, for most types of epilepsy (there are a couple of exceptions), EEGs can only confirm the diagnosis if you actually have a seizure while the EEG is being recorded – and seizures do not usually happen to order! Other limitations are that about 2% of people who do not have epilepsy have EEGs that do not look normal (we do not know why). Add to these limitations the fact that movements (even just opening and closing the eyes, or sucking and chewing) can show up on the recording, and you can see why interpreting EEGs correctly needs so much expertise.

What sort of thing are doctors looking for on EEG recordings?

They are looking for the out-of-the-ordinary brainwave patterns (called 'seizure discharges') which show that the electrical signals in the brain are not being sent correctly. The shapes of the discharges and how frequently they occur during the recording provide information about the type of seizure and where it starts from. Often, helpful information can be obtained from a recording, even though no seizure has occurred. The most useful recordings, however, are those that record actual seizures.

Figure 2.1 shows an example of a normal EEG recording (the outline of the head in the figure shows where the electrodes were placed). The brainwave patterns are symmetrical and

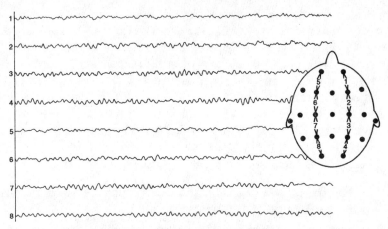

Figure 2.1 Normal EEG recording.

regular and show the electrical activity that goes on in the brain all the time.

Figure 2.2 shows an EEG pattern called 'spike and slow wave'. As it occurs in all the lines on the recording, it indicates a generalized seizure – an absence seizure in this particular example. There is more information about both generalized seizures and absence seizures in Chapter 1. EEGs of absence seizures typically show a pattern of three spike and slow wave discharges each second. Technically this is described as 3 Hz or 3 cycles/second spike and slow wave activity. This is an ictal pattern, i.e. it only appears when a seizure is taking place, and between seizures the EEG pattern appears normal. If you are thought to have absence seizures, then 99% of the time it is possible to bring one on by encouraging you to hyperventilate (overbreathe, i.e. breathe much faster and more deeply than normal). If this is done while the EEG is being recorded, then the typical EEG pattern we have just described will be absolute confirmation of the diagnosis. Absence seizures are very rare in adults, but it is an excellent seizure type for use when the doctor is explaining the EEG and how it works.

Figure 2.3 provides an example of why the information provided by an EEG cannot be used on its own. A spike and slow wave pattern appears again, but this time only on some of the lines

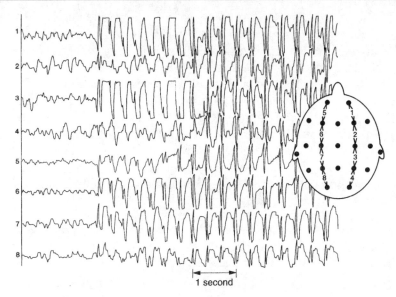

Figure 2.2 EEG recording of an absence seizure showing spike and slow wave pattern.

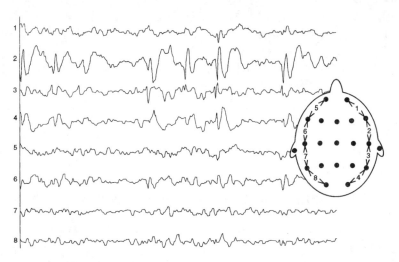

Figure 2.3 EEG recording of a partial seizure starting in the right side of the brain (electrodes 2 and 3).

of the recording. This pattern is both ictal and interictal, and indicates a partial seizure – in this example one starting in the right side of the brain. However, there is no way of telling from the recording whether it is a simple partial seizure or a complex one. The specialist also needs to know exactly what happened during a seizure in order to make a definite diagnosis. For example, if you had some twitching on the left side of the body (remember that the right side of the brain controls the left side of the body) but you remained fully conscious, then this would suggest a simple partial seizure. If you became confused or behaved in a strange way, then this would indicate an affected level of consciousness, and would suggest a complex partial seizure.

I had my first seizure when I was watching television. When I had my EEG, I was made to look at a flashing light and I had another seizure. What was the point of doing this?

This was to check for photosensitivity. A diagnosis of photo-sensitivity was suggested by the fact that your first seizure occurred when you were watching television, and the stroboscope test (the flashing light used during the EEG, sometimes called a strobe) was used to confirm it. If your body jerked briefly when you were looking at the light, then you had a photoconvulsive response (read more about photosensitivity in *More about seizures* in Chapter 1, and in Chapter 9).

The EEG recording in Figure 2.4 shows what happens to the brainwaves when a photosensitive person looks at a stroboscope. The stroboscope has triggered a generalized irregular spike and slow wave discharge (see above). The line below the EEG indicates the stroboscope frequency – in this example it is flashing 12–14 times a second. Technically speaking, it has a frequency of 12–14 cycles/second or 12–14 Hz.

I have already been to out-patients for one EEG, and now been told that I have to have another one. Surely the results will just be the same as the first time, so why do they need to repeat it?

A routine EEG in the out-patients' department of a hospital takes somewhere between 30–90 minutes, and it does have its

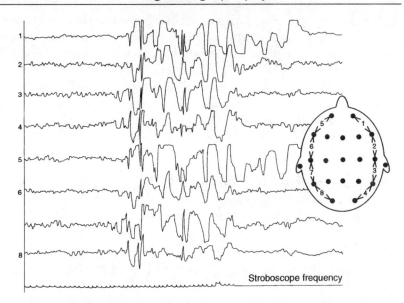

Figure 2.4 EEG recording showing what happens when a photo-sensitive person looks at a stroboscope.

limitations. One important limitation is that it is rare for a seizure to actually occur during an EEG, and interictal EEGs, i.e. those recorded between seizures, often appear normal.

These problems can be solved using a variety of specialized EEG techniques (they are discussed in the rest of this section) and it may be that you are going to have one of these tests next time. The results of your second EEG may well provide different and more informative results than the first one. It is quite usual for EEGs to be repeated until enough evidence has been collected for a specialist to be able to confirm a particular type of seizure or identify a specific epilepsy syndrome.

I was asked to make sure that I stayed awake for some time before I went to the clinic for my EEG. Why wouldn't they let me sleep?

It sounds as if you were going to have a sleep-deprived EEG, perhaps because your routine EEG had appeared normal.

Reducing the normal or full amount of sleep can cause changes in the electrical signals in the brain (it is rare for it to provoke a seizure). These changes would not be seen in a routine EEG, but when they appear after sleep deprivation they may provide important evidence to support a diagnosis of epilepsy. Sleep deprivation also makes it more likely that you will fall asleep naturally during the test, and this is another way that more helpful information can be obtained.

I fell asleep during my EEG, and the hospital staff were very pleased about this as they said it gave them extra information about my epilepsy. Please can you explain why?

There are two possible reasons. The first depends on whether or not you only ever have seizures when you are asleep (nocturnal seizures). The only possible chance of recording a seizure on a routine EEG is for you to sleep during the test! However, the chances of recording nocturnal seizures on a routine EEG are quite low. If your seizures are of this type, then you will probably need one of the specialized EEG techniques – ambulatory monitoring and video EEG – which are more suitable for recording nocturnal seizures, and these are discussed in the answers to the next two questions.

The second and perhaps more important reason is that brainwaves change dramatically during sleep – this happens to everyone, not just people with epilepsy. Research has shown that sleep can activate or unmask out-of-the-ordinary brainwave patterns (discharges). In particular, being asleep can enhance the interictal patterns on the EEG recording, i.e. make the brainwave patterns between seizures more obvious, which means that they provide more information and give the specialist extra clues to help in making a diagnosis of a particular type of seizure or epilepsy syndrome. From this point of view, the most important time is the initial stage of falling asleep, when you are just 'drifting off', as it is during this period that the discharges are most likely to be recorded. Do not worry if you do not have a seizure during the recording – this activity will still show up on the EEG.

I only ever have seizures in my sleep, so the specialist wants me to have a night-time EEG. Do I have to stay in hospital for this, or can I have it at home?

It will depend on the facilities available at your local hospital. A night-time EEG can be carried out at home using a technique called ambulatory monitoring (described in the answer to the next question). If you live far away from the hospital, you will probably need to stay overnight.

What is ambulatory monitoring?

Ambulatory monitoring is a portable type of EEG – it literally means 'EEG monitoring while walking about'. It allows the brainwaves to be recorded continuously over anything from several hours to a few days, a much longer period of time than a routine EEG. The aim is to collect as much evidence as possible to help with the diagnosis. The longer time period makes it more likely that a seizure will be recorded, and the portable equipment means that the test is taking place during your normal everyday activities, rather than in the strange surroundings of a hospital. It is particularly useful for those who have frequent or nocturnal (sleep) seizures.

In ambulatory monitoring, electrodes are attached to the head just as in a routine EEG. The electrodes are then connected to a recorder which is about the size of a personal cassette player and which is worn in just the same way, either around the waist or over the shoulder. The brainwaves are continuously recorded onto the cassette in the recorder. At the end of the test, the tape from the cassette is analysed with specialized computer equipment. This converts the magnetic signals on the tape back to a standard EEG tracing, ready to be interpreted by a specialist.

The specialist isn't sure that I have epilepsy; he thinks that there may be some other reason for the seizures. He wants to do a video EEG. How will this help him decide if I have epilepsy or not?

The test you are going to have is called *videotelemetry* (telemetry literally means 'measurement from a distance'). It uses a video camera linked to an EEG machine, which will allow simultaneous recording of what you are doing and the electrical activity in the brain (the brainwaves). When the videotape is played back, one half of the screen will show you and the other half the EEG recording, which explains the alternative name for this test – 'split screen EEG'. This means that the clinical evidence (what is actually happening) and the electrical evidence in the EEG recording can be looked at together.

Videotelemetry is very helpful in making an accurate diagnosis of epilepsy. There are a number of other conditions which are not epilepsy but which can produce episodes or attacks resembling an epileptic seizure (see above). It is also possible for someone to have epilepsy but for a routine EEG to look normal. The direct comparison of a seizure, and its EEG that videotelemetry allows, provides a solution for these diagnostic problems. If the videocamera records you having one of your attacks but the EEG is normal, then it is highly likely, but not impossible, that you do not have epilepsy and the specialist knows to look for another cause for the condition. If, instead, the EEG shows a pattern typical of epilepsy, then the diagnosis of epilepsy is confirmed.

Another advantage of videotelemetry is that you can be observed over periods of time – several days if it is thought necessary – which means that it is more likely that a seizure will be recorded. The camera acts as the eyewitness (see above) with the added advantage of the simultaneous EEG recording. This makes it a very useful tool in the classification of epilepsy, as well as in accurate diagnosis. Unfortunately the equipment needed is extremely expensive, and so the test is only available in a limited number of hospitals. It is often used in people who are being considered for surgical treatment of their epilepsy.

Scans

What is a brain scan?

A painless and completely harmless way of producing clear and

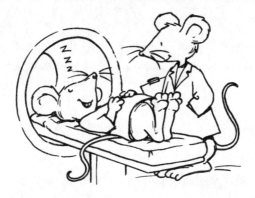

detailed pictures of the brain. The two main types are CT and MRI.

- A CT scan uses X-rays to produce images of the brain which are then fed into a computer. The computer reconstructs these images into 'slices' – pictures of cross-sections of the brain. When these pictures are viewed in the correct order, they build up a picture of the whole brain. CT stands for computed tomography. It is also referred to as CAT scanning (computer-assisted tomography or computed axial tomography).

- Instead of X-rays, MRI uses magnetism: MRI stands for magnetic resonance imaging. The pictures of the brain it produces are similar to those produced by CT scanning, but are much more detailed. For example, a CT scan is an appropriate initial investigation to exclude the possibility of a brain tumour (a rare cause of epilepsy), but less sensitive than MRI in detecting very small brain lesions (abnormalities), particularly within the frontal and temporal lobes (see Figure 1.2 in Chapter 1).

A person having a brain scan will notice little difference between the two types – they both involve lying still within a hollow cylinder at the centre of the scanning machine.

CT and MRI scanning both show the structure of the brain.

Newer type of scans called SPECT scanning (SPECT stands for single photon emission computed tomography) and PET scanning (PET stands for positron emission tomography) also provide information about how the brain is functioning. In the future these types of scan may prove helpful in understanding the classification and causes of epilepsy, but at present their use is limited to research.

Should everybody with epilepsy have a brain scan?

Yes, most people with epilepsy do require one, apart from those with primary idiopathic generalized epilepsies, e.g. typical absence epilepsy or juvenile myoclonic epilepsy (see *Types of epilepsy* in Chapter 1).

A scan can be useful if there is a possibility that the epilepsy has been caused by something actually going wrong with the structure of the brain – perhaps the brain never developed properly, or has been injured or damaged, or has been affected in some other way. The specialist will probably already be suspicious that this may have happened, as there will be other indications as well as epilepsy. For example, there may be other neurological abnormalities or disorders.

The specialist said that the scans were fine. Does this mean that I do not have epilepsy?

No, not necessarily, as the majority of people with epilepsy have normal scans. Scans cannot be used to diagnose epilepsy, but they may be helpful in revealing an underlying cause, or confirming that no such cause exists. In most people diagnosed as having epilepsy, no specific cause for it will be found (see *Possible causes* in Chapter 1).

A brain scan may sometimes have to be repeated, although fortunately this is a rare occurrence. A repeat scan is more likely to be necessary for those whose seizure type has changed or in whom seizure control is poor, and whose first scan was a CT scan done many years ago. Any repeat brain scan will almost certainly be the more detailed MRI scan.

I have read in the paper that MRI scans can diagnose epilepsy. Is this true? We haven't got an MRI scanner near us, so should I ask our doctor to send me elsewhere for one?

The diagnosis of epilepsy is always a clinical diagnosis (see *How do they know it's epilepsy?* earlier in this chapter for the reasons). MRI therefore cannot diagnose epilepsy. However, it is a useful investigation in some groups with epilepsy and may reveal an underlying cause for a person's seizures.

The decision to carry out MRI depends upon the clinical evidence, i.e. what your doctor has observed about you and the information that you have provided about yourself. Not everybody who has epilepsy needs such a scan, and you may well be in this group. We would suggest that you arrange to talk it through with your doctor to find out if you really need MRI. This would be preferable to putting on pressure for what may be an unnecessary test.

I'm frightened that my epilepsy means that I may have a brain tumour. I am going to have a scan – does this mean my specialist thinks so too?

Not necessarily. Scans can show whether or not someone has a brain tumour, but they can also show other things as well, so the fact that you are going to have a scan does not automatically mean that the specialist suspects a tumour. It is important to remember that brain tumours are rarely a cause of epilepsy. As we do not know the details of your epilepsy, we would suggest that you talk your fears over with the specialist, who will be able to explain exactly why you are to have a scan.

3
Treatment

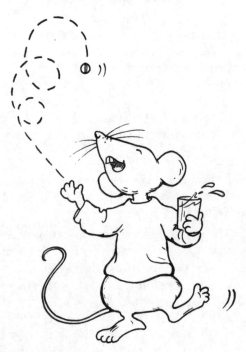

Introduction

The terms 'antiepileptic' and 'anticonvulsant' are often used interchangeably by doctors when they are talking about epilepsy treatments. Both terms mean exactly the same thing. You may also hear doctors talking about a 'drug', 'treatment', 'therapy' or 'medication'; once again these are all interchangeable terms. In

There is a glossary at the end of this book to help you with unfamiliar medical terms.

54

this book we have decided to use the expression 'antiepileptic drug', but this is just our personal choice, and your doctor may prefer another term. Much of this chapter is about these anti-epileptic drugs, as they are the most usual treatment for epilepsy. But we also consider surgery for epilepsy, and look at what place, if any, the complementary therapies have in the care of people with epilepsy.

Does treatment work?

How easy is epilepsy to control?

As you are probably aware, there are many different types of epileptic seizure and many different types of epilepsy (see *Types of epilepsy* in Chapter 1). Fortunately, most types of seizure and most types of epilepsy are fairly easy to control with treatment. This includes being able to stop the seizures for up to two or more years. Overall, about 60–70% of people with epilepsy will have their seizures controlled completely with one antiepileptic drug. In approximately another 10% the epilepsy will be controlled, but only by using a combination of two drugs.

In the remaining 20–30%, the epilepsy is difficult to fully control. It is in this group that antiepileptic drugs may need to be changed to try to find the most suitable drug or drugs, i.e. those which can control as many seizures as possible and without causing side effects. Unfortunately, this may take some time – even many years – to achieve. Occasionally seizures can be controlled for several months but then, for a number of reasons, this control can be lost and the seizures may start again. This could happen either because you are not taking the antiepileptic drugs as prescribed, or because a larger dose may be needed. It may be the result of another illness (see *Practical aspects of drug treatment* later in this chapter) or it may simply be a feature of that particular type of epilepsy.

My seizures are very difficult to control and drug after drug has been used. The hospital doctor just seems to be adding one drug to another. Is it right that I should be taking four antiepileptic drugs?

In the answer to the previous question, we mentioned that seizures can be controlled with a single antiepileptic drug in about 60–70% of all people with epilepsy. Unfortunately, this statistic also means that between 30 and 40% will not have their seizures controlled by just one drug. Sometimes adding another drug (so that you are taking two) will then control the seizures – whichever two drugs are used will be chosen because they work well together. It is very rare for three antiepileptic drugs to work where two have not, and this should be avoided whenever possible. However, it is a very individual response to a drug and it is worth trying different drugs in turn.

Nobody should be treated with four antiepileptic drugs, not only because four drugs will be ineffective and unhelpful, but also because there will be an increased chance of side effects. It is very important that you talk to your hospital doctor about your concerns.

Does epilepsy ever just go away?

Yes, epilepsy does sometimes 'go away' of its own accord. The technical term for this is 'spontaneous remission'. It means that you will stop having seizures and will be able to stop taking antiepileptic drugs. However, it only happens in certain types of epilepsy and it is not that easy to predict, or even to know exactly when the epilepsy has 'gone away'.

Two types of epilepsy where the seizures usually do stop of their own accord are typical absence epilepsy of childhood and BREC (benign rolandic epilepsy of childhood). Seizures will stop by puberty in about 70–75% of children with typical absence epilepsy. In the case of BREC it is thought that all seizures will eventually stop in every child that has it and the drugs used to treat it can then be withdrawn. This is also often around puberty (13–16 years of age), but may be earlier.

Can epilepsy treatment ever be stopped?

Sometimes. As doctors cannot predict exactly when seizures will stop and the epilepsy will have gone into spontaneous remission, it is difficult to know for how long antiepileptic drugs should be taken before they can be withdrawn. Most doctors would advise that if you have been receiving treatment and have had no seizures for five years, then the drug can be gradually withdrawn. Any antiepileptic drug must be withdrawn or reduced gradually over three to six months before stopping it altogether. Stopping taking treatment suddenly can be dangerous and could lead to a condition called status epilepticus (an emergency which is discussed further in Chapter 4).

There is about a 40% chance that seizures will return after treatment is stopped, but this will depend on the type of seizures and the type of epilepsy that has been experienced in the past. If it does happen, it usually does so within a few weeks or months of the drug being withdrawn, but it may not happen for one or even more years. If the seizures do return, they are likely to be of the same type as those that occurred before.

Antiepileptic drugs

Why do antiepileptic drugs have two names?

It is not just antiepileptic drugs which have two names – nearly all drugs do. The first is the generic (the chemical or scientific) name, which is given to the drug when it is first developed. The second is the brand (or trade) name, decided by the pharmaceutical company which makes the drug. Sometimes a drug has more than one brand name, which means that it is produced by more than one company, each of which has given it a different brand name. Generic names are usually written with a small first letter and brand names with a capital first letter.

It can be useful to know the generic names of your antiepileptic drugs as well as the brand names, particularly if you are going abroad (there is more about obtaining drugs overseas in *Medical care abroad* in Chapter 8). Brand names can vary from country to country, but the generic names of drugs are internationally standardized and will be recognized by pharmacists in any part of the world where the drug is available. Generic names must, by law, be printed somewhere on the original container (although they may appear in very small print). Table 3.1 lists the brand and generic names of the most commonly used antiepileptic drugs.

The whole subject of drug names is further complicated by the age of the drugs, i.e. how long it has been since a drug was first produced. Pharmaceutical companies patent the drugs that they develop, and so newer drugs, i.e. those still under patent protection, are only available as the brand name product. They still have a generic name, but they cannot be sold as a generic product. On the other hand, drugs which have been available for a very long

Table 3.1 Brand and generic names of antiepileptic drugs

Brand name	Generic name
Ativan	lorazepam
Convulex	valproic acid
Diamox	acetazolamide
Diazemuls	diazepam
Epanutin	phenytoin
Epilim	sodium valproate
Epilim Chrono	sodium valproate
Frisium	clobazam
Gabatril	tiagabine
Lamictal	lamotrigine
Mysoline	primidone
Neurontin	gabapentin
Nootropil	piracetam
Rectubes	diazepam (as rectal tube only)
Rivotril	clonazepam
Sabril	vigabatrin
Stesolid	diazepam (as rectal tube only)
Tegretol	carbamazepine
Tegretol Retard	carbamazepine
Topamax	topiramate
Valium	diazepam
Zarontin	ethosuximide

time, e.g. phenobarbitone, which first became available in 1912, may only be available under their generic names.

This seems a good place to mention two other very old drugs which are available only as generic products, both of which are still in occasional use today. The first is paraldehyde which is used *only* to stop prolonged seizures or convulsions including status epilepticus (see *Status epilepticus* in Chapter 4). It is effective but it has a strong smell which some people may find a little unpleasant. The second drug is called bromide, and it was in fact the first ever drug used to treat epilepsy (it was discovered in 1880). It has a number of side effects, some of which may be very unpleasant, and it is very rarely used – only in a few specialist epilepsy centres and in very specialized circumstances.

Are there any real differences between branded drugs and their generic equivalents?

The actual drug is the same, whether it is a branded version or a generic one, and both versions should have the same effect in controlling seizures. It is important to remember this, as the products may look very different. For example, the generic version of a particular drug may be available only as a plain white tablet or capsule or as an unflavoured liquid, while the branded product may be a coloured tablet or capsule or a more pleasantly flavoured liquid.

Occasionally there may be a difference between the generic and the branded product in the way in which the tablet, capsule or liquid has been manufactured. Because of this, if a prescription is changed from the generic drug to the brand name drug (or vice versa), then sometimes the frequency of seizures may change (either increase or decrease) or some side effects may develop. It is therefore important to continue with whichever version was first prescribed – it does not matter whether this was the generic drug or the branded drug, just as long as all future prescriptions use the same name.

Generic drugs are usually less expensive than branded drugs, so doctors are often encouraged to prescribe a generic version, if one is available, to keep National Health Service costs down. This price difference will not matter to you, as people with epilepsy do not have to pay NHS prescription charges (see *Finance* in Chapter 7).

I went to my first epilepsy group meeting the other day, and people there were talking about the different types of drugs. I was surprised to learn that the same drug can be available in lots of different forms – as a tablet or a capsule or a liquid and so on. Why?

Most of the antiepileptic drugs come in two or three different forms (also called preparations, formulations or formats). The choice of formulations means that it should be possible for everyone to find a version of their antiepileptic drug which is both convenient and easy to swallow. For example, someone who has difficulty swallowing a whole tablet may find it easier to take a liquid version of the same drug, while someone who takes a midday dose might prefer tablets or capsules as they are easier to carry. There are four common formulations of antiepileptic drugs.

- *Tablets.* Also called pills, these can either be swallowed whole, chewed or crushed. Others can be dissolved in water or fruit juice which is then drunk – these tablets are called dispersible tablets. Some tablets have a special coating: these are known as 'enteric-coated' tablets. The reason for this is that some anti-epileptic drugs can irritate the stomach which can produce some discomfort, including diarrhoea. The enteric coating reduces the chance of this happening ('enteric' comes from the Greek word *enteron* which means gut or intestine).
- *Capsules.* These can be either swallowed whole or sometimes (depending on the particular antiepileptic drug) opened up, and the contents inside emptied out and taken with fruit juice or food.
- *Liquids.* These are often flavoured, and some are available in sugar-free formulations to protect the teeth.
- *Powders.* These are taken dissolved in water, fruit juice or even milk.

Exactly which of these will be available depends on the particular drug, as not all antiepileptic drugs are available in all formulations. For example, some drugs will not be available as capsules, while others will not be available as a powder. Your doctor will know what formulations are available for any particular antiepileptic drug that you are prescribed. It is important to realize that, generally speaking, the drug will do the same job just as effectively, no matter what the formulation.

The British Epilepsy Association (address in Appendix 1) produces a colour poster showing the shapes and colours of the most commonly-prescribed tablets and capsules. The poster also includes other information about these drugs, such as their brand and generic names, the packaging they come in, and the other formulations available. This should enable you to recognize readily your antiepileptic drug/s.

Are all antiepileptic drugs designed to be swallowed or can they be given in other ways?

Regular antiepileptic medication is always given orally (by mouth) and is designed to be swallowed. However, other ways of giving some of the drugs can be used in special circumstances, for example in an emergency.

One formulation of one particular antiepileptic drug is a solution designed to be given into the rectum (the back passage, also referred to as the anus). The generic name of this drug is diazepam, the brand names are Stesolid and Rectubes and they come in a small tube with a nozzle which is inserted into the rectum.

Stesolid and Rectubes are not used on a regular, daily basis but are only given in an emergency when someone has a seizure which lasts for more than a few minutes. Clearly a drug cannot be given by mouth during a seizure as the person will be unable to swallow, but giving the drug into the rectum is effective because it is well absorbed into the blood stream from there. People only need to learn when and how to use rectal diazepam if a relation has epilepsy that is firstly difficult to control and secondly likely to lead to frequent and long seizures.

The other antiepileptic drug available in a rectal solution is paraldehyde, which is *never* given by mouth. Paraldehyde is only used to stop prolonged seizures and never given on a regular daily basis.

There are also some antiepileptic drugs which can be given by injection or intravenously (into a vein). These injections are usually given only in hospital, again in an emergency situation, to try and stop a seizure which has gone on for too long.

Can you reassure me that the newer antiepileptic drugs are really safe to take?

This is a little difficult to answer but we would say yes – probably! All new antiepileptic drugs are thoroughly tested. However, the particular 'licence' (the permit which sets out how a drug should be prescribed) is different for children and adults. The licence only becomes the same for both groups when a drug has been around and available for many years.

At the moment there is a lot of research going on into finding and manufacturing new antiepileptic drugs. The five most recent ones which have been used are vigabatrin (Sabril), lamotrigine (Lamictal), gabapentin (Neurontin), topiramate (Topamax) and tiagabine (Gabatril). Many more drugs are currently being researched and developed and will probably become available in the next three to five years.

There is a difference between the 'older' and 'newer' anti-epileptic drugs. The newer ones have been designed and made specifically to treat epilepsy, whereas the older ones were often first intended for the treatment of other conditions, but then also proved useful as antiepileptics. This targeting of the newer drugs means that they tend to have fewer serious side effects than the older drugs, and could therefore in one sense be said to be 'safer'. However, because they are new and have not been around for all that long, not so much is known about their longer term effects. An example of discovering some things later is the present investigations into whether vigabatrin causes 'tunnel vision'. If proven this will affect usage of this antiepileptic very significantly.

Side effects

Do all the antiepileptic drugs have side effects?

All drugs can cause side effects, even the ones we take for granted such as aspirin and paracetamol, and this is also true for the antiepileptic drugs. The 'older' antiepileptic drugs such as phenobarbitone and phenytoin, both of which were in use before World War II, usually cause more frequent and more severe side effects than the 'newer' ones such as lamotrigine and gabapentin, which have come into use within the last 10 years. Sodium valproate and carbamazepine – drugs first used in the 1960s and 1970s – usually have fewer side effects than the 'older' drugs but may have one or two more than the 'newer' ones!

What are the side effects? Is there anything that makes them more likely to happen?

Because the antiepileptic drugs work on or act in the brain to control the seizures, which start in the brain, they may also cause side effects which affect the brain. Such side effects may include:

- drowsiness
- lethargy (a feeling of tiredness)
- dizziness
- nausea (feeling sick)
- a change in appetite (usually, but not always, an increase), and
- sometimes difficulties with coordination, mood or behaviour.

Some drugs can be associated with extremely rare but serious side effects which may affect the skin, liver or bone marrow (the bone marrow is an essential organ of the body, important in producing all the different blood cells).

Side effects are more likely to occur if an antiepileptic drug is started at a high dose and increased too rapidly. They are also more common when someone is taking two or more antiepileptic drugs at the same time. Fortunately most people need only take one or, occasionally, two antiepileptic drugs to control their seizures. Taking three or more drugs hardly ever results in better seizure control, but nearly always causes more side effects.

How can we know when something is a side effect of drugs and not a new or a different illness?

It is important to ask your doctor (the GP or the hospital specialist) about any side effects, how common or rare they may be, and what you should look out for. Some doctors provide written information sheets on the antiepileptic drugs, including details on any side effects and how to recognize them.

Side effects may be either easy or difficult to recognize, depending, obviously, on what the side effect is and on the person affected. For example, if the side effect is a skin rash or some loss of hair then it will be easier to recognize than if it is only a feeling of sickness (nausea) or a loss of appetite. It may be harder still to recognize side effects in very young children or in people who have learning or communication difficulties: they may be unable to describe what is happening to them and how they are feeling. In these circumstances it can occasionally be helpful to measure the exact amount of antiepileptic drug in the blood to see whether or not the person is getting too much of it.

Should everybody have regular blood tests to monitor their drug treatment?

No, this is not necessary. A blood test can be used to measure the precise amount of an antiepileptic drug in the blood, but it is important to realize that the vast majority of people taking such drugs do not need to have these blood levels measured. The levels only need to be measured in the following situations:

- if the doctor thinks that a person is not taking or is not being given the drug(s);
- if someone has an episode of status epilepticus (see *Status epilepticus* in Chapter 4);
- if someone is being treated with phenytoin, as the metabolism (breakdown) of this drug in the body is complicated;
- if someone has moderate to severe learning or language difficulties and so may not be able to either complain of or describe possible side effects;
- to see by how much a drug dose could be increased.

I have been told that antiepileptic drugs can cause behaviour problems. Is this true?

Behavioural problems tend to occur particularly in people (often children) with learning difficulties and epilepsy. Some of the older drugs, such as the barbiturates, can make this behaviour worse.

My husband's memory seems to have got worse recently; what may be causing this?

Quite a number of people with epilepsy complain about their memory getting worse.

If your husband's memory is genuinely worse, it may be due to a number of reasons. It could be his seizures, especially if they are frequent and long. It may be that he is having some sub-clinical epileptic activity, i.e. activity that cannot be seen externally. You do not say which type of seizures he has, but if he is one of the few adults that continue with absence seizures into adulthood it might be these, purely because he is missing what people say to him.

The older antiepileptic drugs can cause memory problems, especially the barbiturates and phenytoin. As yet, it is thought that the new antiepileptics launched since 1989 may not cause the same problems, especially lamotrigine and gabapentin so, if his doctor thinks it is relevant, a change of drug might be an option.

If the drugs seem to be causing side effects, should I just stop taking them?

No, this would be a very dangerous thing to do. It is very important that antiepileptic drugs are never stopped abruptly – even if you think that the drug is not working or is causing side effects.

If an antiepileptic drug is stopped suddenly it may cause a very prolonged seizure or series of seizures called status epilepticus. This is a medical emergency and may sometimes cause serious problems – it is discussed in more detail in Chapter 4. The most common cause of status epilepticus in all people with epilepsy is suddenly stopping their drug treatment. Any anti-epileptic drug must be withdrawn or reduced gradually, before stopping it altogether, and this process should take at least three to six months. The *only* situation in which an antiepileptic drug can be stopped suddenly is if you are an in-patient on a hospital ward.

None of the drugs used to treat my epilepsy has worked and the side effects of some of them have made me unwell. Should I ask my doctor about not using any drugs at all for a time?

There are a very small number of people in whom antiepileptic drugs just do not work and unfortunately it does sound as if you may be one of them. You are also quite right in saying that some of these drugs can have unpleasant side effects. It is entirely reasonable for you to think that there is thus no point in using any of them. However, you need to remember that your epilepsy could in fact be much worse if you take no treatment at all. On the other hand, it is also possible that, on no treatment, seizures will be no different and you may feel better. If you would like to take yourself off drugs, then you must discuss this with your doctor first and the drugs *must be stopped gradually*. Antiepileptic drugs must be withdrawn gradually over three to six months before stopping them altogether. Stopping taking treatment suddenly can be dangerous and could lead to a condition called status epilepticus (an emergency which is discussed further in Chapter 4).

Practical aspects of drug treatment

I went 10 months without having a seizure, then caught some bug that was going around at work, became ill and now my seizures have come back. Why did they start up again – was it anything to do with being ill?

Quite possibly. People with epilepsy often have periods of remission from their seizures such as you have described. If seizures return during an illness it is possible that an increase in body temperature (a fever) may well be the triggering factor.

If you had gastrointestinal or metabolic problems (causing diarrhoea or vomiting), then these may have reduced the amount of antiepileptic drug absorbed from the stomach and gut. This reduced absorption would in turn have resulted in reduced efficacy, meaning that the drugs would not have been working as well as usual, and because of this further seizures could occur. Fever can also precipitate seizures.

Obviously it is not uncommon for people to have a 'tummy-bug' or gastroenteritis, with diarrhoea and vomiting. If someone with epilepsy vomits within one or two hours of taking a dose of an antiepileptic drug, then the dose can be repeated. If vomiting occurs three or more hours following a dose, then the drug will already have been absorbed from the stomach into the blood stream and there will be no need to repeat that dose.

My doctor told me that I have to take my medicine twice a day. I thought it would help me to remember if I take it when I get up in the morning and when I go to bed at night. Will this be all right?

It will depend on your getting-up time and your bedtime! Strictly speaking, taking a drug twice a day means taking it every 12 hours. Although it is a good idea to try and take the medicine at 10–12 hour intervals, this does not mean using a stopwatch to ensure that it is given to the precise minute or second.

Occasionally doctors do not make it absolutely clear as to how many times a day the tablets or medicines should be taken. Fortunately most only need to be taken twice a day. Very few antiepileptic drugs can be taken once a day, whilst a couple of others have to be given three times a day. It is obviously important for you to ask the doctor how many times a day the particular antiepileptic drug must be taken. If a medicine is to be taken three times a day, then it can be a little difficult to plan the timing of the different doses, and it is useful to work backwards from your normal bedtime. For example, if bedtime is 10.00 pm, then a possible routine could be to take the first dose of the day at breakfast time, the second between 3.00 pm and 4.00 pm, and the third and last dose between 9.00 pm and 10.00 pm.

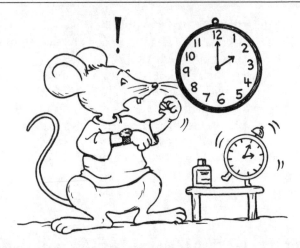

I am rather absent-minded and although I do try to remember to take my antiepileptic drugs when I should, I know that one of these days I'm going to forget and I'm going to miss a dose. Is this going to be very important?

Not if it only happens occasionally. It does not usually matter if one or two doses of an antiepileptic drug are 'missed' or forgotten. As a general rule, if a dose is missed or forgotten but within the next three or four hours you remember that it should have been taken, then it can be taken safely. If you remember the missed dose only five or more hours after it should have been taken, then do not take it. Never, ever, 'double up' any dose because of a previously missed dose. This applies whether you are taking one, two or three antiepileptic drugs.

   As you know that you have a problem with remembering your medication (and you are not alone – it is a very common problem), perhaps you could consider devising some system to help you remember. Try to think of some ideas for a reminder system. You could also consider buying a 'pill reminder', as discussed in the answer to the next question.

How do 'pill reminders' work?

Pill reminders are a practical solution to the very common problem of forgetting to take medication at the right time. They are containers for drugs which enable you to have an adequate supply of your medication handy, particularly if you are away from home, and also to check immediately, by looking at the divisions in the container, whether or not the appropriate dose has been taken. They vary in design, size and sophistication: your pharmacist should be able to show you what is currently available and help you select the most appropriate version. Some of the latest models have a built-in alarm which sounds to remind you that it is time for a tablet, while others even carry a small water supply to help with swallowing it.

I've been asked to keep a record of all my seizures and to bring it with me the next time I go to the hospital. This came up just as I was leaving the clinic so I didn't have time to ask why or exactly what they wanted to know. Please could you explain?

People are often asked to keep a 'diary' of their seizures between clinic visits, as this can provide very useful and important information for the doctor. Keeping such a diary will also save you having to try to remember all the details of your seizures the next time you go to the clinic! The doctor will ask to look at the seizure diary on your next clinic visit, and will use it to assess your response to your antiepileptic drugs. Because of this, it is important that you remember to take the diary with you.

You will need to record when, where and at what time a seizure occurred, how many occurred on a single day, and what precisely happened during the seizure. You could also record any other details that you think might be important, such as any missed doses of drugs. Some of the pharmaceutical companies which manufacture antiepileptic drugs produce free diaries (a typical example is shown in Figure 3.1) and your doctor should be able to provide you with one of these, or tell you where to obtain one. However, an ordinary notebook or exercise book will do just as well.

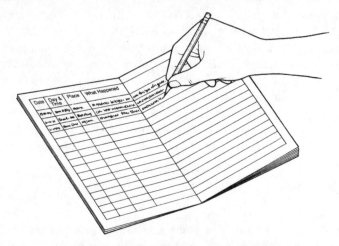

Figure 3.1 A typical seizure diary.

Recently my boyfriend who has epilepsy keeps forgetting to take his medication, in fact sometimes he just refuses to take it, whatever I or his family says. We find this extremely worrying; what on earth can we do?

Your boyfriend's behaviour is not unusual, not that that makes it any the less worrying for you. Non-compliance with treatment (refusing, failing or 'forgetting' to take medication) is very common in people with epilepsy. This refusal or forgetfulness may arise from a lack of understanding about the need to take medication regularly, or it may reflect your boyfriend's inability to accept that he has epilepsy – in this way it is a denial of having the condition.

People with epilepsy need to take over the responsibility for their own condition. They must be given responsibility for taking their own medication, and it is important for you and your boyfriend's family to show him that they have trust and confidence in his ability to take care of himself (easier said than done). However, people need to know exactly why they must take medication and the family is not always best placed to deal with this issue, especially during the rebellious stages of adolescence. Therefore, you may have a crucial role to play. Information and advice may be more acceptable if it comes from a very close friend or a doctor.

Not wanting to take medication may also be due to some of the side effects of the drug(s). This is particularly important for some people who are taking sodium valproate, as this drug can cause hair loss and an increased appetite, resulting in weight gain. If this is what is worrying your boyfriend, then talking to someone outside the family, such as a specialist epilepsy nurse if there is one in your area, or anyone else whom he respects and feels able to trust, may help a lot.

Whatever we suggest, at the end of the day it is up to people with epilepsy themselves whether or not they continue taking medication for their seizures. Family, friends and medical personnel can only do their best to provide accurate advice and information in a sensitive way which will enable these people to make sensible and informed choices.

Surgery

Can surgery be used to treat epilepsy?

It is becoming clear that surgery may actually cure epilepsy. A cure means that after surgery all antiepileptic drugs can gradually be withdrawn and the person never has any more seizures. However, it is very important to understand that only a small percentage, perhaps no more than 4–5%, of all people with epilepsy have epilepsies which would be suitable for surgery and should actually be considered for it.

Are any special tests needed before surgery can be carried out?

Yes, people who may be suitable for surgical treatment will need special tests or investigations to try and find out from exactly where within the brain the epilepsy may be starting. These investigations cannot be done in any hospital: they must be carried out in a specialized epilepsy centre.

The tests will include such things as brain scans (see *Scans* in

Chapter 2) and videotelemetry, which has proved very useful in presurgical evaluation (see **EEGs**, also in Chapter 2). It will also be important to find out where the areas or 'centres' for speech and memory are located in the brain, to try to ensure that any operation will not cause any problems. This is particularly necessary for any operation that might be carried out in the temporal lobe (see Figure 1.2).

How soon after diagnosis should epilepsy surgery be considered?

This is a difficult question to answer, but surgery should certainly be considered in the following situations:

- if the seizures are always partial or focal, i.e. beginning on one side of the brain, occur frequently and do not come under control with two or, at most, three different antiepileptic drugs;
- if the EEG and, more importantly, a brain scan (either a CT scan or, preferably, an MRI scan) shows a single abnormality in just one region of the brain (see **Scans** in Chapter 2).

There are other times when surgery should perhaps be considered, but this will depend on the individual and type of seizure or epilepsy.

It is also becoming clear that if surgery is to be undertaken it should be done sooner rather than later. In the past it was often delayed for many years as it was regarded as a 'treatment of last resort', but today doctors realize that if surgery is necessary and indicated, then the earlier it is performed, the better the outcome. This applies not only to the outcome for the epilepsy but also to relationships with family and friends. It is therefore important to identify as soon as possible those people where the epilepsy is not going to respond to antiepileptic drugs. Age does not matter – surgery for epilepsy can be carried out even in young infants. It can also be carried out on people with learning difficulties. The surgery, however, is expensive and NHS funds are at the moment limited.

Does epilepsy surgery always work?

There are many different types of operation which can be

performed to try and cure or treat epilepsy, and they each have different success rates. The most successful operations are those which are carried out on the temporal lobe (see Figure 1.2). Most operations on the temporal lobe are performed in young adults. Overall, up to 70 or 75% of people who have an operation for temporal lobe epilepsy will be 'cured' and will never have another seizure. Other types of operation do not have such high success rates.

Diet

Do people with epilepsy need any special sort of diet?

No, not usually – but it is important for everyone to eat healthily, not just those with epilepsy. This means choosing meals which are high in fibre, low in fat, and include plenty of fresh fruit and vegetables. It is important that meals are not missed, and strict weight-control diets are to be avoided. If you would like further information about what makes up a sensible diet, you could contact the Health Education Authority (address in Appendix 2) which publishes booklets and leaflets on healthy eating.

A healthy body also needs rest and in some people disturbed sleep or long periods without sleep can trigger seizures. The occasional late night will not make any difference, but it is important to have a regular sleep pattern as part of a healthy lifestyle.

I have heard that it is possible to control seizures by eating a special sort of diet. Please could you tell me more about this?

Attempts have been made to control seizures by changing the diet. The best-known of these is called the 'ketogenic diet'. 'Ketogenic' comes from two other words: *keto* from 'ketones', which are natural substances found in the blood and urine, and formed from the metabolism (breakdown in the body) of fats; and *genic* meaning to produce or make. Thus the diet is literally one which 'makes lots of ketones'.

The ketogenic diet consists mainly of fat, is not very tasty, and therefore is usually not popular! It must be kept to very strictly and a hospital dietician will always need to be involved to ensure that it is worked out properly.

Doctors do not really know how the diet works in controlling seizures and, unfortunately, it does not always work. Even when it does, the effects may only last for a short time – only rarely do they last more than 12 months. Antiepileptic drugs usually have to be continued along with the diet, although occasionally the drugs can be gradually reduced and even withdrawn. The ketogenic diet has a place in the treatment of a few children with difficult epilepsy, but it is not a suitable diet for the majority, and there is little evidence for its successful use in adults.

Complementary therapies

Do doctors disapprove of complementary or alternative medicines?

Before trying to answer this question, we need to make a distinction between medicines or therapies which claim to be 'alternatives' to treatments offered by the medical profession, and those which are 'complementary' and are meant to be used alongside conventional treatments. The use of a complementary therapy should be in addition to, not instead of, your usual antiepileptic drugs. No one should stop taking their normal medication without discussing it with their doctor. This is particularly important with antiepileptic drugs, where sudden withdrawal of treatment can be dangerous (see *Does treatment work?* and *Antiepileptic drugs* earlier in this chapter).

The reservations held by many members of the medical and health professions largely revolve around the fact that very few of these treatments have been subjected to properly controlled research. This means that there is little hard evidence that the treatments really work. If and when they should be used in epilepsy, how effective they are and the precise ways they work have not been fully established.

Doctors may understandably be sceptical about alternative or complementary treatments when people are tempted to stop their usual medication, when the therapies themselves have serious side effects, and when they feel that their patients are being misinformed and persuaded to spend large sums of money which they can ill afford. If these features are not present, most practising doctors will take a neutral or even an encouraging view of complementary therapies and appreciate that, even if the scientific evidence for them is elusive or even non-existent, they may still do some good. Sometimes just the feeling that you are doing something that may help you can be very valuable.

I am keen to try a complementary therapy, because I have read so much about them in the popular magazines. But there seem to be such a lot of different therapies – how do we decide which to try, and how do we find someone to consult?

The answers to the remaining questions in this section will give you some idea of the complementary therapies which have been used by people with epilepsy. Whichever you choose to try, the most important thing is to find a practitioner who is adequately qualified. At the moment there is nothing to prevent someone with minimal training – or even no training at all – setting themselves up in business as a practitioner and treating clients. In untrained hands, complementary therapies can do harm. However, the reputable members of the various complementary therapies are trying hard to improve their own practices and to give the public more information about their qualifications and training.

There are a number of organizations representing com-plementary therapy practitioners: usually each therapy has its own 'governing body' and there are also umbrella organizations trying to improve standards across the whole range of com-plementary treatments. You will find the relevant addresses listed in the *HEA Guide to Complementary Medicine and Therapies* (details in Appendix 2), which also includes suggestions on how to find a suitable practitioner and the questions you should ask before agreeing to a course of treatment. You could also ask at your own GP's surgery or health centre for the names of reputable

local practitioners. Some practices now offer some complementary therapies themselves.

Cost may be another factor that you want to take into consideration. These therapies are not often available on the NHS,
and they can prove expensive.

Whichever therapy you choose, and however you find a practitioner, there are some things which you must remember. You
should talk to your doctor before starting on the chosen therapy,
to make quite sure that it will not interfere or interact in any way
with your medical treatment. You must tell the complementary
practitioner about your epilepsy, and you must continue to take
antiepileptic drugs as usual.

What is aromatherapy? Is it true that it can be used to help people with epilepsy?

Aromatherapy is a complementary therapy involving treatment
with essential oils, which are aromatic (scented) oils extracted
from the roots, flowers or leaves of plants by distillation. Aromatherapy often involves massage, but the oils can also be inhaled
or added to baths.

Interest in aromatherapy has grown rapidly in the general
population over recent years, so it is not surprising that some
people with epilepsy have explored the possibility of using this
therapy to help control their seizures. Some people with epilepsy
use aromatherapy as a form of relaxation, as they believe that
reducing stress in this way in turn reduces the frequency of their
seizures. There are also people with epilepsy who experience an
'aura' before they have a seizure – a warning (usually involving a
strange sensation, feeling, smell or taste) that a seizure is about to
happen. A few of these people have found that smelling a particular aromatherapy oil (usually jasmine, lavender, camomile,
ylang ylang or bergamot) as soon as they notice the aura can
prevent the seizure happening, particularly if they have had
preceding massages.

Unfortunately all the evidence for the use of aromatherapy in
epilepsy is anecdotal – there have been no properly controlled
medical research trials of whether it actually works or not. We
know of only one small and informal hospital study into its use,

and that involved only 50 adults. We need to wait for proper research to be set up and the results published before we can say for certain whether or not aromatherapy can definitely help in epilepsy. We will not have an answer for a number of years.

In the meantime, we can certainly say that aromatherapy is a pleasant means of relaxation, provided that all the precautions we have mentioned elsewhere in this section are followed, e.g. conventional treatment with antiepileptic drugs must be continued. It is particularly important to find a properly qualified aromatherapist: people with epilepsy should avoid those practitioners whose qualifications are in the use of aromatherapy as a beauty treatment rather than as a complementary therapy. Aromatherapists would also recommend that you avoid buying the essential oils available over the counter in health food shops without taking proper advice first, as not only do they vary in quality, but some of them can actually increase seizure frequency (examples include rosemary, sweet fennel, camphor, hyssop and sage) and so should not be used. Evening primrose oil should also be avoided.

What complementary therapies have been tried for epilepsy? Do any of them actually work?

At a guess, probably all of them by some people with epilepsy somewhere in the world! However, apart from those already mentioned earlier in this section, the ones that are most likely to be tried are the following:

- *Acupuncture.* This is a traditional form of Chinese medicine which involves inserting special very fine needles into the skin at particular sites on the body in order to balance the 'life energy' or 'vital force' which the Chinese call *ch'i* or *qi*.
- *Homeopathy.* This therapy is based on the principle that 'like can be cured with like'. The remedies used contain very dilute amounts of a substance which in larger quantities would produce similar symptoms to the illness being treated. Homeopathic doctors believe that illness is caused by imbalances within the body and they concentrate on strengthening the body's natural defences. Homeopathic remedies should only be used after a discussion with both a doctor and a

qualified homeopathic specialist (homeopathy is available through the NHS although the provision is limited).

- *Hypnotherapy.* A person who is hypnotized enters a state of very deep relaxation, during which they are more receptive to suggestions of ways of altering behaviour than they would be in a fully conscious state. While it is most useful in reinforcing good intentions to change bad habits, such as stopping smoking, it can also be helpful in reducing stress and increasing confidence. People with epilepsy need to be 'awoken' slowly after hypnosis and only accredited hypnotists should be consulted.
- *Relaxation.* Some complementary therapies, e.g. massage, encourage relaxation, but it is also possible to learn how to relax consciously at will, either at classes or by listening to special cassette tapes. Relaxation therapy has been shown scientifically to reduce seizure frequency.

The real use of all the complementary therapies that we have described is in aiding relaxation and helping relieve some of the stress and anxiety that may be found in people with epilepsy.

Some people will claim that these complementary therapies are useful in epilepsy, but it is extremely unlikely that any of these methods are effective by themselves: antiepileptic drugs will still be needed. In other words, they really are complementary – they are a complement to, not an alternative to or substitute for, conventional treatment with antiepileptic drugs. But as long as these different treatments do not interact or interfere with conventional treatment, there is no reason why they should not be tried. As already mentioned, it is important to discuss all non-medical treatments with your doctor before embarking on any course of complementary therapy for your seizures.

4

Is it an emergency?

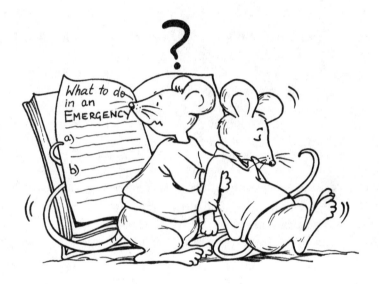

Introduction

Is a seizure an emergency? More often than not, the answer to this question is no. But everyone should know what to do when a seizure occurs (or what not to do, which is equally important), as well as how to recognize an emergency and what to do in those circumstances.

There is a glossary at the end of this book to help you with unfamiliar medical terms.

One situation which is definitely an emergency is *status epilepticus*. Although status epilepticus is rare, when it occurs it is potentially a very serious condition, and so it has its own section at the end of this chapter.

All the types of seizure mentioned in this chapter are explained in more detail in the sections on *Types of epilepsy* and *More about seizures* in Chapter 1.

First aid

Can you give us some general first aid rules for what to do when someone has a seizure?

First aid is not required for most types of seizure, although there are exceptions, including generalized tonic-clonic seizures and complex partial seizures, and these are dealt with below. All seizures should be allowed to run their natural course: recovery times will vary from person to person, and will also depend on the type of seizure. Try not to panic.

My girlfriend wanders in her seizures. What should I do?

People who wander during a seizure usually have complex partial seizures, during which they may behave strangely and they may appear confused. General first aid advice is as follows:

- Be understanding and talk gently and reassuringly to her while the seizure is continuing.
- Only attempt physical contact with her if she appears to be at risk of harming herself, in which case move her gently away from danger.
- If there is no danger, let the seizure take its natural course.

John has different seizure types but what can we do when he has one of his major convulsive seizures? What is safe?

Some general first aid advice for this type of seizure is as follows:

- Aid his breathing and airway by turning him onto his side and, if possible, into the recovery position (shown in Figure 4.1), and loosening any tight clothing.

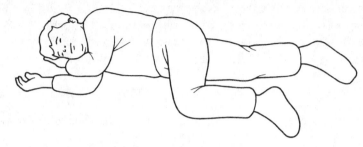

Figure 4.1 Recovery position.

- Protect him from injury by moving furniture or other hard objects out of his way if possible.
- Protect his head from injury, e.g. by putting a cushion, pillow or folded-up sweater or coat underneath it, or by using your hands or arms.
- Do not move him unless he is in immediate danger, e.g. has fallen near a fire or on a staircase.
- Do not leave him alone until he is fully recovered.

One thing you very definitely should **not** do is to attempt to put anything between his teeth. This is not safe, and could cause considerable damage to his teeth. It could also result in you receiving an unpleasant bite.

When his lips go blue, is it dangerous? Do we need to call the doctor?

Blueness around the mouth (called perioral cyanosis) is caused by a low level of oxygen in the blood (see *More about seizures* in Chapter 1). It is usually self-limiting: a pink colour returns rapidly once the seizure has ended and normal oxygen levels have returned. It is not dangerous in itself, and medical help will only be needed if the seizure does not end spontaneously within a few minutes. When to call for help is discussed in the next section in this chapter.

Is it safe to let a person fall asleep after a seizure?

Yes. Most generalized tonic-clonic seizures are followed by a period of sleep, which may last from half an hour up to several hours. This is normal following this type of seizure and is part of the post-ictal phase, i.e. what happens after a seizure. Some people may also fall asleep after a complex partial seizure. Recovery times following seizures vary from person to person, but as long they are not left unattended and are kept under observation, it is safe to let them sleep for however long they need.

Should all carers learn how to give rectal diazepam (Stesolid, Rectubes) as a first aid measure?

No. Carers only need to learn when and how to use rectal diazepam if their relative or partner has epilepsy which is firstly difficult to control and secondly likely to lead to frequent and long seizures. If this is the case, then you should be taught about rectal diazepam; if it is not, then you are unlikely ever to need it. You could check with your doctor about this if you are at all concerned.

Stesolid and Rectubes are the brand names for two formulations of one particular antiepileptic drug whose generic name is diazepam. It is a solution which comes in a small tube to be inserted into a person's rectum (the back passage, also referred to as the anus). Clearly a drug cannot be given by mouth during a seizure as the person will be unable to swallow, but giving the drug into the rectum is effective because it is well absorbed into the blood stream from there.

Calling an ambulance

Should my work colleagues call the GP every time I have a seizure?

In most cases the answer to this question is no, but there will be exceptions. We would suggest that you talk it over and decide between you if and when they should call the local surgery or health centre. There are circumstances when calling for emergency help is necessary (which will mean dialling 999 for an ambulance rather than ringing your GP) and these are listed in the answer to the next question.

If I have a seizure or a series of seizures, at what stage should someone call an ambulance?

Emergency medical care should be considered in the following circumstances:

- If a second or third seizure occurs without you regaining consciousness.
- If the convulsive part of the seizure is lasting longer than usual, and certainly if it lasts longer than 10 minutes.
- If you have any injuries that occurred during the seizure, e.g. cuts requiring stitches.
- If the cause of the seizure is uncertain and further investigation is necessary.
- If for any other reason someone is worried or concerned either during or after your seizure.

What happens once the ambulance arrives?

First of all, it is important that whenever possible someone who saw the seizure gives a detailed account to the paramedics or the ambulance crew on their arrival. They will assess the situation and administer emergency first aid should that be necessary. Once in the ambulance, a member of the crew will remain with you until you arrive at the Accident and Emergency Department of the hospital.

Should someone accompany me to the hospital after I have had a seizure?

Yes, if at all possible, for two reasons. The first is that you will obviously feel less scared and worried if you have someone else you know with you. Your friend or colleague or eyewitness should ask the ambulance crew if he/she can travel in the ambulance but, if for some reason this is not possible, then he/she should get to the hospital as soon as possible.

The second reason is that the eyewitness will be needed at the hospital to tell the doctors in the Accident and Emergency Department exactly what happened. It is not essential for eye-witnesses to travel in the ambulance, but the doctors will want to talk to them as soon as possible after they have reached the hospital, so they do need to get there quickly.

What happens when we reach the hospital?

On arrival at the hospital you will be given a thorough medical examination by a doctor. A medical history will be taken, and it is important that a detailed account of the seizure is given to the hospital staff (the importance of eyewitness accounts is explained in *How do they know it's epilepsy?* in Chapter 2).

What happens next depends on whether or not the seizures have stopped. If the seizures are continuing, then emergency medical help will be required: you may be given intravenous antiepileptic drugs such as diazepam. If, on the other hand, the seizure has stopped and a post-ictal condition exists, then you may remain in the hospital for a period of observation. This may be for a few hours, or perhaps overnight, depending upon a number of factors including how well you are, whether there is another medical condition which may have caused the seizure and which needs treating, and your wishes.

Status epilepticus

What is status epilepticus?

The currently internationally accepted definition of status epilepticus is either:

- any seizure lasting for at least 30 minutes; or
- repeated seizures lasting for a total of 30 minutes or longer, from which the person does not regain consciousness between each seizure.

Any type of seizure may develop into status epilepticus, although few do – fortunately it is a rare condition. Generalized tonic-clonic seizures are the most likely to lead to status epilepticus: this is called convulsive status epilepticus, and is the most serious type. The other type is called non-convulsive status epilepticus and may occur in absence epilepsy and with complex partial seizures. It is easy for doctors to recognize convulsive status epilepticus, but non-convulsive absence status and particularly non-convulsive complex partial status may be more difficult to diagnose. EEGs (see Chapter 2) are very important in diagnosing non-convulsive status epilepticus.

Convulsive and non-convulsive status epilepticus are medical and neurological emergencies and need to be treated quickly. If you think that your partner or colleague is in status epilepticus, then call for help immediately, as discussed in the previous section on *Calling an ambulance*.

Can status epilepticus cause brain damage?

Epilepsy rarely causes brain damage. Convulsive status epilepticus (explained earlier in this section) may cause brain damage, but only if it is not treated promptly. The only situation where recurrent generalized or partial seizures may cause brain damage are if either:

- the seizures are so frequent, i.e. happening every few minutes for days at a time, that the person (and the brain) does not recover between seizures; or
- a single seizure (usually a tonic-clonic seizure or convulsion) lasts for more than 60–90 minutes without stopping.

Is status epilepticus life threatening?

It can be, but the risks today are far less than they used to be. About 6% of people with status epilepticus still die these days. It is therefore important to diagnose and treat rapidly. However, today's lower risks do not make status epilepticus any less serious. Convulsive and non-convulsive status epilepticus (defined above) are medical and neurological emergencies, and the outcome depends on the time interval between the seizures beginning and the start of effective treatment. Convulsive status epilepticus may be life-threatening, particularly if it lasts 30 minutes or longer, which is very rare. Non-convulsive status is not life-threatening, but it is still a medical emergency as it can sometimes change into convulsive status. Non-convulsive status occurs when someone has recurrent absence or complex partial seizures without recovering consciousness.

I recently heard someone on the radio talking about SUDEP. What is this?

SUDEP is an abbreviation for something called sudden unexpected death in epilepsy. It is only over the last few years that it has received any publicity and we need further research to explain it better.

It is thought to be the most common form of death during a seizure. At present it is only a guesstimate, but it is thought that about 400 people in the UK die each year from this cause. It tends to occur in people aged between 20 and 40 years who have tonic-clonic or complex partial seizures. The risk of someone dying for this reason does vary immensely between different groups of people, mainly whether people are in remission or not. Basically people who have had their seizures controlled are very unlikely to have another seizure that may cause an unexpected death, whereas those who have frequent seizures may have a risk as high as 1 in 200 people. The risk also increases if someone is not compliant with the medication.

The cause of death is still open to argument, but respiratory problems are suggested as a likely cause and may explain why most people die at night whilst alone.

It is important that people are aware that death can occur in epileptic seizures, but it is just as important, if not more so, to realise that it is very rare for it to happen.

5
Feelings, families and friends

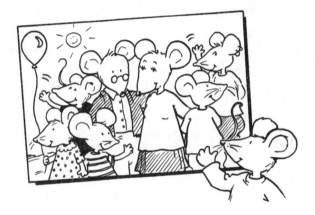

Introduction

Being told that you have epilepsy is bound to be a shock, and many thoughts and feelings will flash through your mind. Different people will react in different ways: some will feel worried and depressed, others angry. Some people will find the diagnosis a relief as they have been imagining something much worse, others

There is a glossary at the end of this book to help you with unfamiliar medical terms.

will want to blot out the news completely in the hope that it will just go away. These are all very natural reactions, as are your worries about how your family and friends will respond when you tell them about it. There is some more help also in Chapter 10.

Coming to terms with epilepsy

Are conditions such as epilepsy really discussed more openly these days? My GP seems to be suggesting that it would be a good idea for me to talk to other people more about my epilepsy. I really don't know where to start.

We think conditions such as epilepsy are talked about more openly these days. They are certainly discussed more openly in the media than was the case a few years ago.

When it comes to talking on a more personal level, then everyone is different. Some people will find it easy to talk about it, but for many families this is not the case. There are any number of reasons for this reluctance, ranging from not wanting to accept the diagnosis to simple embarrassment at discussing personal feelings. Of course it takes time to adjust to being told that you have epilepsy but, in our experience, being able to talk about it can help, even when sharing your feelings is difficult.

Finding out more about epilepsy from as many sources as possible is a good way to increase your family's confidence in discussing it. Your own particular experiences will of course be unique to you, but you will find that many of them will be similar to those of others. The various epilepsy associations are good starting places for finding out more about epilepsy, and you will find their addresses in Appendix 1.

If you feel it would be helpful to talk to someone outside your family, then you could ask your doctor to put you in touch with other people with epilepsy, or perhaps with an experienced counsellor – these counsellors can be found at many of the specialist epilepsy centres. If there is an epilepsy specialist nurse in your area then that would be another source of help, information and support.

My partner is very upset about my epilepsy and won't help at all; he seems to just want to ignore it. What can I do?

Everyone in a family needs time to come to terms with epilepsy, and often the last person to accept the diagnosis is the one closest to you. The reasons why can be many, but you may need his help and support, both now and in the future. It is in everyone's interests that all members of the family are pulling in the same direction.

He should be encouraged to talk about his feelings as soon as possible. Talking to him about your own feelings and how much you value his support might be a possible starting point.

Epilepsy scares me. Will this fear ever go away?

Being told that you have epilepsy can be frightening, especially if you know little about it. Learning more about epilepsy can help, as can talking about your fears and worries.

Above all you need to give yourself time to come to terms with the diagnosis. It is a bit like a bereavement – you have lost something (your complete good health) and you need to give yourself the opportunity to grieve for your loss and accept it. The fear will gradually subside as you gain experience and confidence. You may never lose it completely, but it will no longer be at the forefront of your mind all the time.

I worry a lot about my epilepsy, but I find it difficult to talk about it to my partner. Is there anyone else I can talk to?

Your doctor or epilepsy specialist nurse (if you have one) might be able to help. Some GP practices also now provide counselling services. The British Epilepsy Association has a confidential Helpline with a freephone number. Their experienced Advice and Information Officers could be of assistance (see Appendix 1). The various epilepsy associations also have local branches where you could meet other people with epilepsy.

If we extend 'talking to' to include 'writing to', then a penfriend with epilepsy would give you the opportunity to share your concerns with someone who has similar problems. You may find one through the penfriends page of *Epilepsy Today*, the magazine of the BEA. These days we are all well aware of the dangers of releasing our names and addresses to complete strangers, which is why the BEA operates a box number system for potential penfriends. A potential penfriend will not have to know your identity until you are quite happy that the replies are genuine and that you have made a suitable choice.

If you have access to the Internet, then you could join in one of the various epilepsy discussion and support groups that exist in cyberspace – the fact that you can be completely anonymous there might encourage you to communicate when it is difficult to do so in person. The BEA now has its own Website.

My wife rarely goes out since her epilepsy was diagnosed; she says she is terrified of stepping outside the front door. What can I do to help?

You will need to try and find out exactly why she does not want to go out. It may not be her epilepsy, but if it is there are a number of reasons she may be frightened. The most common are the fear of having a seizure in the street or a shop, or perhaps what may happen in a seizure (for example, being incontinent), or the first aid she may suffer.

We know that you are not meant to suffer during first aid, but she may be frightened of someone breaking her teeth or injuring her in some other way or perhaps she does not want to finish up in casualty because of people calling for an ambulance. In the case of her seizures, it may be that she feels embarrassed about what may happen.

What you can do to help is complex, but a good starting point as we keep mentioning is to talk about her concerns. You may then be able to encourage her to go out more in company before the major challenge of on her own. Other people, like her GP, specialist nurse or hospital doctor, may also be able to help. There are specialist services for people with a fear of going out (*agoraphobia*), for whatever reason, and her GP should be able to put you in touch with them locally.

Do you think a person with epilepsy should be described as that, or as an 'epileptic'? I dislike it when I hear someone refer to me as an 'epileptic', but I don't want to make any unnecessary fuss about it.

You now have a diagnosis of epilepsy, but is this a reason to use any labels? Depending on how your friends treat you, you are the same person that you were before and having any sort of label will not help. You and your epilepsy will both be very individual and should be treated as such, not labelled.

As you will have gathered, in our opinion, labels like 'epileptic' are very unhelpful, although unfortunately they are still used frequently, including by some professionals who should know better. However, informing people calmly and politely of your feelings about this can hardly be considered to be making a fuss.

Family feelings

Now I have epilepsy, my brother is worried that he may develop it. Is this likely?

His fear is a very common response. You can be reassured that there is no reason why your brother's health status should change, as the chances of him developing epilepsy are very small. Keep everything in perspective: learning more about epilepsy may help with this, as knowing the facts may enable him to cope with his fears.

My youngest brother hates my epilepsy, because he says his friends no longer want to come to our house. How can I help him overcome this?

Your brother's friends may be frightened because they do not understand what epilepsy is, and he may be reinforcing this by expressing negative views about it to them because he may still feel frightened himself. Reassurance should help – perhaps you could explain to him what epilepsy is and how little there would be to do if you had a seizure (see *First aid* in Chapter 4). Your brother's self-confidence could be lower than usual and this will take time to recover, so some positive conversations about epilepsy are probably required. When your brother feels reassured, then you could encourage him to talk positively about your epilepsy to his friends.

I feel unable to cope with my partner's seizures. What should I do?

First aid for seizures is usually easy and information is freely available from the various epilepsy associations (addresses in Appendix 1). Read this or similar information from other sources (see *First aid* in Chapter 4, for example). You could also try to help manage a seizure if you are present with others, as this should help you build up your confidence to deal with any that happen if you are alone with her.

These suggestions should help on a practical level, but you should talk about your real concerns with local people who can help you, such as your doctor or epilepsy specialist nurse, if you have one.

Outside the family

My husband and I are trying to work out how to tell other people about my diagnosis. At the moment we can't even decide who needs to know. Can you help us make up our minds?

Almost everyone will have to share news about health issues at some time in their lives, and news about epilepsy is no different. If you are worried about people's reactions, then you will probably be pleasantly surprised. Ask the people you tell what they would like to know: each response will be different, but they are more likely to be interested and concerned rather than discomforted. If you do come across a negative reaction, it will probably be caused by ignorance, and you should be able to overcome it by providing information about epilepsy and talking about it in a positive way.

One reason why you need to tell your family and friends is that you may need their help if you are to carry on with your life as

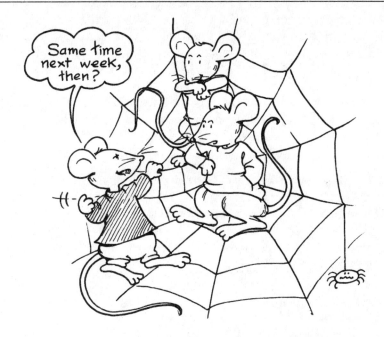

before. If you do not tell them, they may be imagining problems far worse than epilepsy, if they had been worrying about your health.

When it comes to people that you know less well, then only you can decide what is appropriate. You should tell people with whom you will be working, in case you have a seizure at work and need to arrange time off for hospital appointments and so on (see Chapter 6). You may want to tell your neighbours, even if they are only acquaintances rather than friends. Whatever you decide, take a positive approach in the telling: being positive yourself invites a positive reaction.

Since we told our friends about my epilepsy, there is one couple that we hardly seem to see any more. We think it is because they are frightened of it. We want to carry on as normal, so what can we do? Can we really still expect them to make us welcome?

People can be apprehensive about epilepsy for many different reasons, so you will need to try and find out what is really bothering your friends and then provide them with the information that will help to reassure them. After your conversation, give them some time to absorb what you have told them and adjust to it, and then we would hope that they would be as welcoming as before. You might discover that your worries about them were unfounded, and that they thought they were behaving in a helpful way. Perhaps they wanted you to have time to adjust to the diagnosis without being worried by social calls, or they may have simply not known how to talk to you about it.

All the people who know about my epilepsy have been very sympathetic, but my partner and I feel that they don't really understand that we just want to lead an ordinary life. This applies not just to our friends, but also to some of the medical staff that we meet. How can we make them understand what we want?

In other words, you don't want sympathy but you do want empathy. Some people will treat you sympathetically thinking that this is helpful, and you will need to try to explain to them just what it is that you want. Tell them that you intend to live life as before and that constructive help to do this would be more than welcome. Only you can know what you consider to be constructive help.

You may also have to discuss this issue with the medical staff. Some professionals will still provide you with a list of things you should not do now that epilepsy has been diagnosed. This is a negative attitude, and it would be more useful for you to find out the facts about why you can still carry on with your usual activities rather than why you cannot.

6
Employment

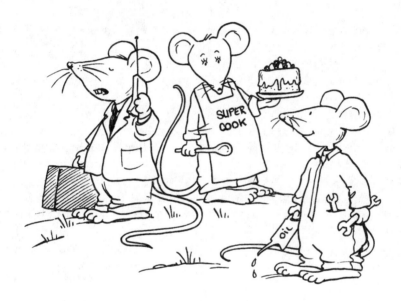

Introduction

Work is so important in people's lives, it is not surprising that there are many specific questions to ask. Many of our answers are equally applicable inside the school or college environment. Anyone close to a person with epilepsy will need to know something about the condition, and in most cases

There is a glossary at the end of this book to help you with unfamiliar medical terms.

the information they need will be very similar to that outlined
here.

Teaching the employers

**Does my employer need to know about my epilepsy?
Wouldn't it be easier if I kept the news to myself?**

If you want to have a safe, active and successful career, then yes,
your employer does need to know. If you find it difficult to talk
about your epilepsy then it might be easier for you not to mention
it, but it would certainly not be better – colleagues' ignorance
could lead to you being inadvertently put at risk.

Most people worry about an employer's and their colleagues'
reaction to a diagnosis of epilepsy. We cannot predict what
response you will get, but it will probably depend how much these
people already know about epilepsy. Some will be knowledgeable
and very helpful, others may be less so. If you can take a positive
attitude when you break the news, then you are more likely to get
a positive response. We discuss whom and what to tell in the
answers to the next few questions.

If you are asked about your health on an application form or at
an interview and do not disclose that you have epilepsy, then at
any time in the future you can be dismissed for not revealing the
information. At the moment there is no legal protection for
applicants refused a job on account of their health (even if you
could discover that that was the real reason), and almost none for
employees dismissed because of their health record.

If you think that this is unfair, then we agree with you. In other
countries, e.g. for example the USA, employers cannot ask such
questions at the application stage. If they ask them after offering
someone a job, then only an occupational health specialist and not
the employer is allowed to make the decision as to whether that
person is medically fit for the position. Such a system is far fairer
than the current situation in this country, where decisions about
fitness for employment are made by people without appropriate

qualifications – an arrangement which often leads to unnecessary discrimination.

The Disability Discrimination Act (DDA) should, in theory, prevent discrimination in employment. How it will work in practice it is perhaps too soon to know, and even if it proves effective, discrimination will still be allowed if the employer can show 'good reason' for it. Companies employing fewer than 20 people are exempt from the provisions of the Act, as are organizations such as the police and the Fire Service. One person with epilepsy has won a court case for unfair dismissal under this new Act, so this could be used as a precedent in future cases.

All this leaves you and other people like you in a difficult position, and we cannot offer an easy answer to the problem. You will need to decide whether to keep quiet about your epilepsy and risk dismissal at some future time, or whether you should tell potential employers about it in a way that convinces them that it will not affect your ability to do the job. We would strongly recommend the latter option (see also the next question.)

Generally speaking, the more information and knowledge employers and colleagues have, the more understanding they will be – and this will help not just you, but all people with epilepsy.

If I reveal my epilepsy on a health questionnaire, by perhaps ticking a relevant box, how much more should I outline in a covering letter?

It is an excellent idea to enclose a covering letter, and it should cover things that outline why your epilepsy should not be a problem. You need to concentrate on things that may make your seizures predictable. These commonly would be:

- being seizure-free;
- having an 'aura' (warning) of your seizures;
- having a pattern to your seizures – perhaps they only happen when you are asleep, or in the first hour after waking up;
- having a specific 'trigger' for your seizures – perhaps watching television, for example (photosensitivity is covered in Chapter 9).

These things mean that you know when your seizures may occur and that you should have time to sit or lie down, or even better, that the seizures will never occur at work.

Your letter must be positive, strongly selling your abilities and stating why your epilepsy is not a problem.

Some health questions are asked at interviews. How should I respond?

We feel that you should reveal your epilepsy and, as discussed in the previous question, explain why it will not be a problem for the job that you are being interviewed for. It is important to consider those aspects of your epilepsy mentioned in the question above.

At a recent interview, an employer said that they could not employ me because they did not have any medical personnel on site. Is this fair?

It certainly is not and may not be justifiable under the DDA. You do not need medical personnel for first aid (covered in Chapter 4) and next time you must point this out quite forcefully.

I realize that I must tell my employer, but I'm not sure where to start. Who would be the best person to contact?

Different employers will have different policies about this, which will probably depend at least partly on the size of the firm. Your first point of contact is most likely to be your immediate boss, but in a larger firm it might be someone with special responsibility for employee welfare or human resources. If you were given some literature about the firm when you started there, then this might tell you who the correct person is, or you could perhaps ask the receptionist for this information. Another approach could be to start by telling a colleague whom you already know quite well, and take advice on what to do next.

Wherever you start, it is important to emphasize that someone you work with regularly should be aware of your epilepsy. Whoever you choose to tell should either know what to do if a seizure occurs or whom to call for help.

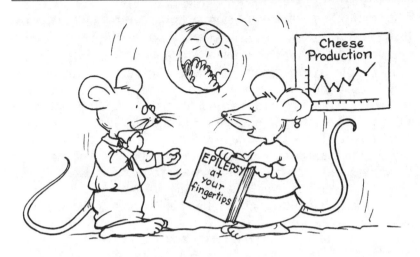

Exactly what should I tell my employer?

Do you mean about epilepsy in general or your epilepsy in particular? What you have to tell them about epilepsy in general will depend on how much they already know: you may find them very knowledgeable, or you may have to start with the basics.

When it comes to your own epilepsy, then you will need to tell them:

- what your seizures look like;
- if you get any warning (aura) of a seizure;
- how long the seizures last;
- how long a rest you need after a seizure;
- what first aid may be required;
- how many seizures you are having each week or month;
- if there is a pattern to the seizures or if you know of anything which makes them more likely to happen;
- what action you would like the staff to take if there is an emergency.

The epilepsy associations (see Appendix 1) also have some helpful literature that you could offer them.

Why are so few employers sympathetic towards people with epilepsy?

Not all employers are unsympathetic. Epilepsy is so common that many people involved in management and staff recruitment have friends or family members who have had seizures, and these employers are unlikely to discriminate against other people with epilepsy. There are also companies and organizations with genuine equal opportunities recruitment policies, unfortunately fewer in number than those who claim to have such policies but somehow never put them into effect. In many ways you have to take pot luck: some employers are sympathetic, some are not and it is virtually impossible to find out which employer is in which group. One way of getting more information about your local companies is to contact the Employment Service (the address will be in your phone book) as they have a scheme that recognizes employers who show a positive attitude towards people with medical conditions.

After many interviews, I have still not been offered a job. Is this because of my epilepsy?

Epilepsy might be the reason, but you should not automatically assume that this is the case. Today's job market is very competitive, so applicants need very good qualifications and the ability to sell themselves to prospective employers. It may be that you are not doing yourself justice: information of how best to present a CV and coaching in interview skills might be more useful than worrying about your epilepsy. However, you will also need to work out the best way of telling prospective employers about your epilepsy. Also, having the knowledge and self-confidence to correct any inaccurate ideas about epilepsy that they may have will be useful.

My employers are trying to be very helpful about my epilepsy, but it is very obvious that they actually know little about it. As my diagnosis is still very recent, I am still learning about it myself, and I find that I can't always answer their questions! Where can I get some help?

The various epilepsy associations produce information packs, and any of these would make a good starting point. Contact them at the addresses given in Appendix 1 for further details. You could also arrange for someone – perhaps an epilepsy specialist nurse or someone from a local epilepsy group –to contact your employer to explain about epilepsy and answer questions. If you cannot find a suitable person yourself, then one of the associations may be able to suggest someone in your area.

What action should I take if I have problems in coping with my work, or if my employer is not very understanding?

It is becoming less common, but it is still not unusual for an employer to be difficult when someone develops epilepsy. If you have problems we would suggest that you attempt to provide your employer with a little bit of information about epilepsy generally and your epilepsy in particular, emphasizing why your condition should not be a problem for the job that you presently do. Most employers, provided with the correct understandable information, are reasonably accommodating. Problems may occur with fellow employees, and a similar line of providing information may be beneficial.

Getting on at work

What type of career should I be aiming for because of my epilepsy?

Jobs barred by law are covered in a later question and, except for these, people with epilepsy are involved in every career imaginable. You should not rule out anything until you know more about how your epilepsy will respond to treatment. More important is to consider your qualifications and experience.

Sometimes, doctors will say that people with epilepsy can do anything except for jobs at heights and on machinery. This advice is very non-specific and probably not helpful. What is a machine? Is it guarded? Is a height referred to, guarded? Does the person have predicable or unpredictable seizures?

If your seizures are controlled or prove to be predictable, most careers will be open to you, and it is important that you obtain any relevant qualifications that you need for whatever job you choose. If your seizures are frequent and unpredictable, then your choice will probably be less and you will have to find out more about particular work environments, but many jobs should still be open to you.

Are there any specialist employment advisory services for people with epilepsy?

Yes. If you are still at college, then you should get in touch with your local careers advisory service. Contacting them can be a little confusing now that the service has been privatized, but your college should be able to tell you what to do. If they cannot help, then ask your local TEC (Training and Enterprise Council) for help, or you may find something listed under 'Careers Service' in your local phone book. Your local library may also be able to help with information.

Once you have made contact with the service, you should find that there is someone there who specializes in advising people with medical conditions. It might be a particular individual who deals mainly with such people, but in some areas all the members of staff are now trained to provide this type of advice. Because these people inevitably have to deal with a wide range of medical conditions, their knowledge of epilepsy may be limited, but if you approach them early enough, before unfortunate career choices are made, they should be able to offer constructive advice.

If you have already left college, then you can approach the Employment Service for advice (the number will be in your phone book). Their local Placing, Assessment and Counselling Team (PACT) will include people who specialize in helping adults with a medical condition find work, as well as disability employment advisers who offer a wide range of services.

If someone is allowed to drive after one year free of seizures, why are they not allowed to enter professions such as teaching and nursing after the same time span?

In some cases they are: it all depends on the school of nursing or the teacher training institution. Quite a number of people with epilepsy are nurses or teachers, but they have sometimes found it difficult to get through the system. It is currently recommended that people with epilepsy should have been seizure-free for one year before they start teacher training, but some institutions will take a candidate's individual circumstances into account before making a decision about admission to the course. Each school of nursing seems to set its own rules, which can be confusing. If someone is committed to either profession there is no reason for them not to press ahead, but they must realize that some people will attempt to put barriers in their way.

There is a section on *Driving* in Chapter 7.

Are any jobs legally barred to people with epilepsy?

Yes, some are. They include occupations where having a seizure could be a genuine safety hazard, for example the armed forces, the Fire Service, driving a train or ambulance, or piloting a commercial aircraft. The various epilepsy associations produce excellent leaflets on employment that explain these restrictions and they can also help with up-to-date information on employment law and regulations, as the entry rules for certain jobs do keep changing (for example, organizations such as the police will now consider employing people with epilepsy whereas in certain jobs they would not).

Is a job that requires a driving licence a sensible career choice?

We can only give a general answer to this question, as we do not know the details of your epilepsy, how well it is controlled and how it will affect you in the future. Medical research shows that the longer epilepsy has been controlled, the less likely it is to return. If you have now been seizure-free for some time, e.g. for three years or more, then such a job would be a perfectly reasonable choice. If you have only been seizure-free for a year, then, although you will be able to hold a licence, it would be sensible for you to wait a little longer before starting on a career where driving was crucial. There is a section on *Driving* in Chapter 7.

My husband is a qualified accountant but he is unable to drive, so he is off work. Is there any way he could be helped to work from home?

The employment service do have various schemes where financial help may be provided in order for people to work from home. You should find out the address and telephone number of your local job centre and attempt to make an appointment to see either one of the 'front line' staff or the Disablement Employment Advisor. Any of these staff should be able to inform you about the grants available in your local area. The grants tend to be for equipment. As an example, if you were wanting information technology to help you work from home, they may be able to help.

Will I find it easier to get a job if I register as disabled?

The new Disability Discrimination Act has brought registering as disabled for employment purposes to an end, so this option is no longer be open to you. There was in any case little evidence that registering as disabled helped anyone's employment prospects; instead it often seemed to have a negative effect. Most people with epilepsy quite rightly chose not to register.

I am worried that I may not progress at work. I seem to miss out on promotion and am accused of low output. Is this anything to do with my epilepsy?

There are various reasons why this may be happening, not all of them connected with epilepsy. It is sometimes easy for people to blame their epilepsy for lack of promotion, but it may mean that other causes are being ignored.

If you think that your epilepsy is the cause, then the following are the most likely explanations you need to consider:

- staff (and you?) assuming that you will not achieve because of your epilepsy;
- frequent seizures of any type;
- damage to the brain, however minimal, which may affect your ability to remember things, concentrate etc.;

● side effects of antiepileptic drugs (although this is not usually
the most common cause) – most commonly drowsiness, poor
memory, poor concentration.

You need to discuss all these factors with your employers in an
attempt to find out which appears to be the most important. You
may find that more than one is a problem. Hopefully you will be
able to solve any problems easily, but for some you may need the
help of your doctor or another professional.

If you do have genuine problems coping at work you will
need to look for the reasons why. Is it really your epilepsy
or is there some other reason. If it is your epilepsy, it will
probably be one of the factors mentioned earlier in this answer
that is causing the problem, and you should discuss this with
your hospital consultant or general practitioner to see whether
changes can be made to your medication regime to improve
matters. There could be other reasons like stress at work which is
making your seizures worse or perhaps overtiredness. It is only
you who can decide where the problems are and, after identifying
them, you need to take positive steps to overcome them. This will
probably best be achieved by discussing your worries with all
concerned.

What effects might my diagnosis have on my job security?

It is difficult to answer this question as you do not say what type of
job you already have. For most people, the diagnosis should not
cause too many problems, especially if the seizures are controlled
quickly without side effects from medication.

It is a good idea to discuss your diagnosis with your employer
and to take into account the work environment that you are
presently in. The environment will probably not need changing,
but it is sensible to consider whether problems might occur.

If you have a job which involves a great deal of driving your
diagnosis will have a major effect, because you will have to forfeit
your licence and inform the DVLA.

The effect therefore for each individual will always be very
varied, depending on the particular job involved.

I've got epilepsy and I've had no problems at my current work. I've now been offered a new job, but I will have to have a medical before they confirm the offer – it's not just me, they make everyone have one. Do I have to tell them about my epilepsy?

Whether to reveal epilepsy or not to an employer is covered in the first section of this chapter and similar issues do apply here. However, have you revealed your epilepsy to your present employer? If the answer is yes and you have been successful in your present post, you could use this information very positively, saying that your epilepsy has not been a problem and therefore will not be for the new post. If the answer is no then things are more difficult, because you have no positive feedback available.

Either way, ethically, you should be telling the person doing the medical about your epilepsy, so things are out in the open. Perhaps, you could find out who the information is shown to and, if it is only seen by the medical staff, this may give you more confidence to reveal your epilepsy.

What help is there if an employer wants to sack me because of my epilepsy?

If you are in a Union, you could try them first. You could also get in touch with the British Epilepsy Association (address in Appendix 1) or your local Disablement Employment Advisor based at your local job centre for advice. They may be able to tell you how best to proceed in your particular case.

We can only answer generally, but crucially, how many discussions have you had personally with management? It is always better to negotiate yourself, if this is still an option. If the worst is looking likely, you could always go to an industrial tribunal. The Disability Discrimination Act may help here. One lady recently won her case for unfair dismissal under this Act and was awarded compensation.

I'm about to take up a job abroad. What should I do about my epilepsy drugs and my medical supervision while I'm there?

As you don't say where you are going, this is difficult to answer. If we assume that you are going to work in a developed country, there should not be any problems unless you are taking one of the newer antiepileptics (vigabatrin, lamotrigine, gabapentin, topiramate or tiagabine). These drugs are now available in many developed countries, but it does vary greatly from country to country, so check with your doctor or the one of the epilepsy charities (addresses in Appendix 1).

In many cases your medical supervision will be on a private basis, so you need to check what the costs might be and whether the costs can be avoided, say by agreements between Britain and the country you are living in. Your doctor may be able to advise on this, or you could try enquiring about relevant contact points in your local post office. The company for whom you are going to work may also have an employee health scheme.

If you are going to work in less developed countries, say Africa, you could have many more problems. Some countries do not have regular supplies of even the old antiepileptic drugs (such as phenytoin, carbamazepine, sodium valproate) so you would need to check very closely, with the company you are working for, the details of the overall health care provided by them.

I am taking some university exams this year. What happens if I have a seizure when I am in the middle of them – how will it affect my results?

There are no definite rules, and policy does vary between the examination boards, so the advice we can give here must be very general. Depending on how far you are through the examination and whether you are capable of continuing after the seizure, then the examination board may be willing to take into account the fact that you did have a seizure during the examination. You may need to appeal to the board outlining the exact facts, and this would certainly be worth doing should it unfortunately prove necessary. It will be easier for the board to come to a decision if the course concerned also has a major continuous assessment section.

Have you considered contacting the relevant board well in advance of your exams to find out exactly what their attitude would be? It may also be helpful to have a letter from your doctor explaining the situation, particularly if your seizures are not well controlled.

Will I able to get the same insurance at work as my colleagues?

Employers sometimes use insurance as an excuse for not employing people with epilepsy, but you should not accept this. Employer's Liability Insurance is what is needed and all the major insurance companies in the UK have undertaken to insure people with disabilities in the workplace. They class epilepsy as a disability, therefore there is cover available, usually at the same cost as for anyone else.

For those not able to work

Our son integrated well at college but, because of his severe epilepsy and slow progress academically, should he consider sheltered accommodation and/or sheltered employment when he leaves college?

These are issues many parents of young adults with severe epilepsy have to face. To find out what will be best in his case, you will need to discuss your worries and opinions with him.

In the case of employment, he will probably need to get advice from the disablement employment adviser and the PACT service mentioned earlier. With their advice, a sensible future in employment can probably be planned. You should not accept a conclusion of sheltered employment unless it is absolutely necessary.

Concerning accommodation, you should get in contact with the Social Services department of your local authority. They will be able to tell you about local facilities, and they also have a duty to provide residential care for all those who 'by reason of age, illness, disability or other circumstances are in need of care and attention which is not otherwise available to them'. They will need to make an assessment of your son's needs so that they can identify the most appropriate residential placement for him.

You may also be concerned about how the costs of future care will affect your finances. This is another reason for seeking specialist advice sooner rather than later. The earlier you can start saving, the easier it will be to meet any financial targets you need to set yourself.

I have been told that I am unlikely to get a job, so will I still receive the normal state benefits?

There is a difference between being unlikely to get a job and being considered incapable of working because of disability or severe ill-health, and it is not clear from your question which of these applies to you. We can give a general answer here, but would also suggest that you obtain more detailed information either from the various epilepsy associations (addresses in Appendix 1) or from the Benefits Agency's freephone Benefit Enquiry Line (listed under Benefits Agency in your local phone book).

In general terms then, if you are capable of working and are actively seeking work (although unable to find a job), then you are entitled to the usual benefits for the unemployed under the usual conditions. If you are assessed as being incapable of work, you should be able to claim Severe Disablement Allowance (a weekly cash benefit paid to people who do not have enough National Insurance contributions to qualify for Incapacity Benefit) if you fulfil any of the following criteria:

- you are at least 16 and under 65 years of age;
- you have been continuously incapable of work for 196 days and are still incapable;
- you satisfy the residence conditions of the UK;
- you qualify under one of four conditions:
  - you are entitled to a non-contributory pension;
  - you were incapable of work on or before your 20th birthday;
  - you can be passported to the test of 100% disablement; or you are assessed as 75% disabled.

As qualifying for some benefits can often bring automatic entitlement to others, it would be well worth you getting specific advice for your particular circumstances.

7
Practical concerns

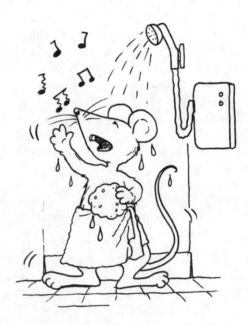

Introduction

This chapter is intended to answer many of the questions that affect daily living when you have epilepsy. It covers a broad sweep of topics, from baths to benefits and from doors to dentists. The common link is that they are all 'how to' concerns with practical answers.

There is a glossary at the end of this book to help you with unfamiliar medical terms.

Safety in the home

My partner and I keep arguing about how many changes we need to make in our home now that we have been told that she has epilepsy. I know things have to be safe, but we still want to have a nice, normal home. Is this possible?

Yes, of course. Without knowing more about your partner and her epilepsy we can only speak generally, but in most cases the precautions you will need to take will only be those you would make to keep any home safe. They should not have to affect the comfort of your home or be obvious to anyone else. For example, you might need to rehang bathroom and lavatory doors so that they open outwards – then the door will not be blocked if your partner falls behind it – but who will notice the difference?

It is a rare person who has never had an accident of some sort at home. We should all probably take more care about home safety. RoSPA (the Royal Society for the Prevention of Accidents – address in Appendix 1) produces information leaflets on the subject, which you might find useful. When you know that your home is reasonably safe anyway, then you can go on to consider any extra changes, if any, you may need to make to allow for your partner's epilepsy.

Should I continue to do all my cooking now that I have been diagnosed as having epilepsy?

In all but the most severe cases of epilepsy the answer is yes, but there are certain basic precautions you should take. A cooker guard would be sensible, and pan handles should always be turned inwards towards the cooker, not left sticking out into the room. Remember to take plates to pans rather than carry saucepans containing boiling liquids. If you can afford one, a microwave oven would be a safer option than a conventional cooker.

What is the safest form of heating for our house now that I have epilepsy?

All heating is potentially dangerous, but it is usually easy to protect yourself from the dangers whether or not you have epilepsy. Instead of spending a fortune on changing your heating system, why don't you just spend a little on fire or radiator guards? However, it would be best to avoid free-standing heaters.

Many of the inner doors in our house are mainly glass. Do we have to change them for solid doors?

Not necessarily. It might be safer in case you have a seizure and fall into and break the glass panel but, if you like the doors that you have, then you could replace the original panels with safety glass. There are recommended standards for such glass and your local glass merchant should be able to advise you – you might discover that you already have safety glass fitted.

My partner has very frequent seizures involving falling and I am worried about the dangers that our furniture presents. What can we do?

Some families in your situation have moved as much furniture as possible away from the middle of the room, especially in rooms used regularly where the furniture is solid and has sharp edges. Some pad their furniture with soft materials like foam rubber, but others think that this alters the appearance of the home too much. It is quite easy to hide padding on chairs, tables and bed bases under covers or valances, more difficult to hide it on items such as cupboards and wardrobes. Other options are to replace free-standing pieces with fitted units – for example, replacing a wardrobe and chest of drawers in a bedroom with a wall-to-wall built-in system, so getting rid of any sharp edges.

Exactly how you change your present home environment, if at all, is your choice and will obviously depend on how much space you have and how much you want to spend. However, we would suggest that next time you buy something new, take your partner's safety into account when considering its design.

I have been told that having a bath may be dangerous. Is this true?

Possibly, but we cannot say definitely without knowing more about your epilepsy. The risks are obviously less for those whose seizures are either predictable or well-controlled by treatment. A few people with epilepsy do die from drowning each year while taking a bath, but as no specific records of this are kept, we do not know the exact numbers and so cannot put it into perspective. As supervision while you are having a bath is obviously unsatisfactory, try to make sure that you only bath when someone else is in the house and leave the bathroom door unlocked. The door should open outwards so that it cannot be blocked if you fall behind it.

A shower would be far preferable, as it is safer – it is possible to sustain an injury in a shower, but the chances are far less. Try to avoid shower bases with high surrounding lips, choose a shower fitting with an efficient heat control, i.e. one which cannot be turned to the warmest setting accidentally, and make sure that any shower screens are made from safety glass or plastic.

Driving

Will I be allowed to learn to drive?

Yes, if you have had no seizures at all in the last 12 months or have only had seizures in your sleep during the last three years (these times run backwards from the date on which your driving licence takes effect). You must tell the DVLA (the Driver and Vehicle Licensing Agency) about your epilepsy when you apply for the licence. If you contact the DVLA's Drivers' Medical Unit (address in Appendix 1), they will send you details of exactly what information they need, but basically it is just a matter of completing a form and providing them with the name of your doctor. With your permission, they will then contact the doctor for a medical report that you are fit to drive.

When you pass your test, you will be given a full licence with a limited life, usually for one year at first and then for two periods of three years. Once you have held a full licence and been seizure-free for seven years, you will be issued with the standard licence that lasts to the age of 70. If you do have another seizure at any time, whatever the cause and however minor, then you must stop driving and notify the DVLA. Your licence will be withdrawn until you have once again completed the regulation seizure-free period. You will not need to take another driving test to get your licence back.

All these regulations may seem tedious, but the aim is to make driving as safe as possible for everyone. A car out of control is a lethal weapon, and serious accidents can occur in a fraction of a second.

You haven't mentioned medication – do I have to have stopped taking drugs before I learn to drive?

No. It is very important that you continue to take your anti-epileptic drugs as prescribed to prevent a seizure occurring when you get your licence and are driving.

If you and your doctor decide that you no longer need drugs, the DVLA advises that you should stop driving whilst treatment is withdrawn and for six months afterwards. You are not legally bound to do this, but it would be the most sensible course of action. Should you have a seizure either after your medication is withdrawn or because of some other change in treatment, e.g. switching to a different drug, then you will have to stop driving and give up your licence until you have once again been seizure-free for the required time.

If I pass my driving test, will the car insurance cost a lot more?

The answer will depend on your insurance company. Most motor insurance companies now offer cover to people with epilepsy, but some charge a higher premium. Other factors – such as the type of car you own, the area you live in, your claims history and your age – are likely to have far more influence on the price you will have to pay than your epilepsy. You will need to shop around for the best deal, but please ignore any insurance brokers who claim that there is no motor insurance for people with epilepsy, as this is simply not true. If you have any problems, then contact the British Epilepsy Association (address in Appendix 1) as they offer motor insurance through their brokers.

I'd like to buy a motorbike, but will I be able to get a licence?

The licensing position is the same for motorbikes as for cars (as discussed previously) but insurance is another matter. The British Epilepsy Association's motor insurance scheme does not cover motorbikes, and many people with epilepsy have found it difficult to get suitable cover from other companies.

We live on a farm, so can my husband drive on our private land even though he is still having seizures?

It is legally possible for someone without a driving licence to drive on private land, so technically the answer to your question is yes – but are you and he willing to take the risk? Have you considered what would happen if he had an accident? Not only would he risk serious injury, but the costs could be considerable, and you would be very unlikely to be covered by your insurance. If he does decide to drive, then at no time must he go onto a public highway, however small and quiet. He could face a severe fine or even imprisonment for doing so.

I have always wanted to drive a large lorry for a living. Will I be able to do this?

By a large lorry we assume that you mean one for which you would need an LGV (Large Goods Vehicle) licence. You will only be able to obtain such a licence if you have been seizure-free *and* off medication for 10 years *and* a doctor chosen by the DVLA considers you fit to drive. The same regulations apply to PCV (Passenger Carrying Vehicle) licences which allow people to drive buses and coaches. This is quite a recent change in the law and not everyone is aware of it, so if you do qualify please do not be put off by incorrect information.

If you cannot yet qualify for an LGV or PCV licence but do hold an ordinary driving licence, then you will be allowed to drive a light goods vehicle. We would suggest that you contact the British Epilepsy Association's helpline (phone number in Appendix 1) for up-to-date information about the vehicle weight limits involved.

Finance

I have life insurance, which I took out two years ago. Should I tell the company about my recently diagnosed epilepsy? And what if I want to take out other policies in the future?

Yes, you should tell the insurance company, since not telling them could invalidate the policy. As your epilepsy has been diagnosed well after you took out this insurance, you should have no problems, because the company assessed the risks and set the premiums at the time of writing the policy, i.e. when it was first taken out.

Most of the major insurance companies will insure people with epilepsy but they may charge extra for doing so. If you have any problems in the future, contact the British Epilepsy Association (address in Appendix 1). Through their brokers they have many types of insurance available for people with epilepsy (including life, accident, motor vehicle and holiday cover) and they should be able to provide a policy for you.

How the new Disability Discrimination Act will affect insurance provision for people with epilepsy is something that we do not yet know. In theory, the Act will make it against the law for a service provider (and insurance companies are service providers) to make it impossible or unreasonably difficult for anyone to use that service. In practice various exceptions and special conditions will be allowed, so we will just have to wait and see.

Will I be able to get a mortgage?

Quite simply, yes. You may have some problems with the life insurance to cover your mortgage, but it is available. If you do have problems, the British Epilepsy Association will be able to help, through its insurance brokers.

Is a person with epilepsy entitled to any sort of disability allowances or benefits?

Not automatically, as it depends on how severe the epilepsy is. As the vast majority of people with epilepsy respond quickly to treatment, most are not entitled to any disability allowances or benefits. Those who may qualify tend to have very frequent seizures and/or another associated condition.

If you think you may be among those who qualify, you can telephone the Benefits Agency's freephone Benefit Enquiry Line (listed under Benefits Agency in your local phone book) for more information. Your local Citizen's Advice Bureau (again listed in your phone book) may also be able to help, or perhaps one of the epilepsy associations (addresses in Appendix 1). Claiming the correct benefits can be a complicated procedure with many detailed rules to follow, so getting good advice before you start will be invaluable.

If you are in or going into higher education, at some point you should contact your local Education Authority (they will be listed in your local phone book) about the standard maintenance grant. When you speak to them, you could enquire about the additional allowance that is available for disabled students. This extra allowance is related to parental income and is only paid out in very specific circumstances, but if you have other problems as well as epilepsy, or very frequent seizures, then it may be worth asking about it.

My partner has very severe epilepsy and I have to care for him 24 hours a day. Is there any financial help I can get?

You may be able to claim Disability Living Allowance, which is a tax-free benefit for people with disabilities. It has two component parts: the care component which is payable at one of three different rates, and the mobility component payable at two different rates. Each component has a different disability test. The benefit is made payable in the name of the person with epilepsy, not of the parent or carer. If you are successful in claiming either the middle or higher rate care component on behalf of your partner, then you should also be able to claim Invalid Care Allowance for yourself, provided that you spend at least 35 hours a week looking after him. Invalid Care Allowance is taxable.

In the answer to the previous question, we said that claiming the correct benefits could be a complicated procedure – now you know why! You are most likely to succeed in your claim if you get advice from people with previous experience of these applications, so don't hesitate to take advantage of their know-how.

Our company is thinking about starting a pension scheme. Will I be able to join, although I have epilepsy?

Obviously you need to talk to your colleagues who are dealing with setting up the company pension scheme, but you should have no problems. The only possible problem that we can think of is if the pension scheme has a component covering early retirement for health reasons. The insurance company that provides the pension scheme may see epilepsy as a higher risk for this category. You need to check this out and encourage your colleagues to look elsewhere if this is the case.

Is a person over 16 still entitled to free prescriptions?

Yes. If you are staying on in full-time education, then all you will need to do is tick the appropriate box on the back of the prescription form and sign it. If you are leaving school at 16 then you will need an exemption certificate.

To obtain an exemption certificate you first need to get a copy of the Department of Health leaflet P11 (called *NHS Prescriptions – How to get them free*) from your doctor, a chemist's or the Department of Social Security. Fill in form B on the leaflet, ask your doctor to sign it and send it off as directed, and in due course you will receive an exemption certificate. The actual procedure when you hand in your prescription at the chemist's will hardly change at all – it just means ticking a different box on the back of the form.

Exemption certificates currently last for five years, and you will need to renew it at the end of that time by filling in the form again.

Information for carers

We are desperate for a night out, but feel uncomfortable about leaving my elderly mother with a sitter. Are we being overcautious?

Not really. You will need to find a sitter in whom you have complete confidence and, just as importantly, the sitter must be confident about managing your mother's epilepsy. This should be possible, but you will need to talk things over thoroughly with any potential sitters, and provide them with all the information that they may need (you could base it on the list of information given in *Teaching the employers* in Chapter 6). Make sure that the sitter knows where you will be and how to contact you easily if there is a problem. Even better, your mother may have a friend who is willing to sit with her.

Could I get a community care assessment? What is this, and would it really be of any help?

All local authorities have the duty to assess the needs of people who require help with daily living (usually because of age or long-term illness or disability) and then, if found necessary, to provide them with suitable support. The assessment process is called a 'community care assessment', and the amount of care provided will depend on the needs of the person being assessed and the resources available locally.

Whether you will be eligible for help will depend on the severity of your epilepsy and if you have any other medical problems. If you get in touch with your local Social Services department they will give you information about requesting an assessment and on the services they can provide.

Services available through community care mainly involve practical care in the home, e.g. you may be offered help in adapting your home to make it safer or more comfortable, or they may be able to provide an item of special equipment that you need. You may also be offered help with holidays.

My elderly partner needs an immense amount of looking after and I am exhausted. How can I get some sort of break?

The jargon term for this is 'respite care', whether it be a break for a few hours, a whole day, or for long enough for you to have a holiday. Having a break is very important, as you need to be able to recharge your batteries if you are to go on caring for your partner. To find out what is available locally, start by contacting your local Social Services department (or ask the specialist, who may also be able to offer some advice). The department should arrange for someone to visit you to discuss the particular type of respite care that you want, the resources available and any likely cost.

Respite care provision varies considerably from area to area. It may be organized directly by Social Services or by a voluntary agency on their behalf. Your partner may be offered a place in a day centre or day hospital or a residential place in a home; a care attendant to look after your partner in your own home, or care in the private homes of families who have registered with Social Services may also be offered. A useful publication called *Taking a break* (details in Appendix 2) explains these alternatives, and also discusses the fears and concerns that carers may have.

Miscellaneous

What happens if I have a seizure when undergoing dental treatment?

Many people worry about this. Your dentist should know what to do, but for your own peace of mind it would be preferable to make sure that he or she knows all the details (the type of seizure, the medication you are taking and any first aid that may be necessary). Tell the dentist about your epilepsy at your first appointment after diagnosis.

Dental care and treatment for those with epilepsy can be even more important than usual, because some of the drugs, especially phenytoin, can cause gum infections. Good regular cleaning will usually prevent any problems.

Are there advantages in making a private appointment to see a consultant about my epilepsy?

A private appointment will usually get you seen by a consultant much sooner than waiting for an NHS appointment. You will still have to be referred by your doctor. It is useful to ask your doctor to refer you to a consultant with a special interest in epilepsy. After the first appointment you can ask to be transferred to the NHS provided your consultant has an NHS job as well as working privately. Investigations such as a MRI & EEG can be done much quicker privately – usually within a week compared with many months on the NHS – but cost a significant amount of money. A private appointment will also ensure that you only see the consultant, not a junior doctor in training. If you have an insurance policy, it is important to check that any consultations or investigations for your epilepsy will be covered by the policy. Most policies will exclude pre-existing conditions.

I know I am sometimes incontinent when I have seizures in my sleep, and this ruins my bedding. How can I reduce the damage and am I entitled to any financial help?

You can buy waterproof mattress covers, incontinence pads and other forms of protection from a chemist's, but you might like to get some information on what is available before you decide exactly what to purchase. You may have a local Continence Adviser (ask your doctor to refer you), or there are various voluntary organizations which can offer advice – try the Continence Foundation's Helpline or the Disabled Living Foundation (all addresses and telephone numbers are in Appendix 1).

Direct financial help to assist with the costs of incontinence is not available, and what other help you can get varies from area to area. In some areas the Social Services department provides a laundry service. Health Authorities have the power to supply aids such as incontinence pads, disposable drawsheets and protective pants free of charge, but financial constraints mean that some have decided not to provide such aids at all or to limit the quantity supplied.

Should I wear or carry some sort of identification saying that I have epilepsy?

This is a good idea. You have a choice of an identity card or a piece of identification jewellery, and they both have their good and bad points.

A number of organizations recommend identity cards as they can be very useful. They are made of card or plastic and there is room to write in details of your name, address, telephone number, doctor, seizure type and the appropriate first aid. They are available from the various epilepsy associations (addresses in Appendix 1) or your doctor may be able to provide you with one, as some of the pharmaceutical companies issue them free of charge. They have two drawbacks. The first is that people in this country are quite reserved and often will not look through someone's clothes or belongings for such a card. The second is that you have to remember to take the card with you rather than leave it in the clothes you were wearing the previous day, and you obviously run the risk of losing it.

Identification bracelets and necklaces are available from three companies – Golden Key, Medic-Alert and SOS Talisman (the addresses are in Appendix 1). Styles vary: on some you would need to have your details engraved, while others can be unscrewed to reveal a slip of paper containing the relevant information. Many people think that they are preferable to identity cards as they are far more easily seen, more difficult to lose or forget, and by now most of the population knows that they exist and why.

8
Travel and holidays

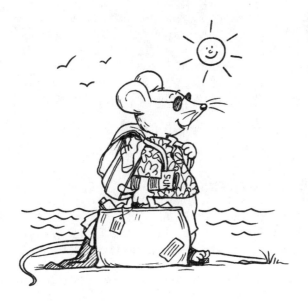

Introduction

We all enjoy being on holiday, but sometimes the organizing needed before we set off is so stressful that we wonder why we are bothering to go at all! When you have epilepsy, then the list of things that you need to remember in your planning becomes a little longer. The suggestions in this chapter are

There is a glossary at the end of this book to help you with unfamiliar medical terms.

intended to provide practical solutions for these additional concerns.

Trains and boats and planes

I've been told that people with epilepsy can obtain a disabled person's railcard. Is this true?

Yes. British Rail originally included people who have continuing seizures, as part of their scheme for disabled passengers. In the medium term, we do not yet know how this scheme will be affected by the current privatization of the railways. At present, however, things are as before. Your nearest main line station will be able to give you information.

Is there a similar scheme for bus travel?

At present there is no national scheme, but similar concessionary fare schemes do exist for local bus travel in some parts of the country. Not every area has such a scheme, but where they exist they are organized by local authorities and/or passenger transport executives, and you should contact them for further information (their addresses should be in your local phone book, or your library may be able to tell you how to contact them).

I hate travelling by sea. Will the stress of this make me have a seizure while we are on the cross-Channel ferry?

Does your epilepsy usually become worse when you are under stress? If your answer is that stress can 'trigger' your seizures, then travelling by sea could pose problems. The problem is the stress, not the sailing, so you could start by trying to find out why you dislike the ferry so much. For example, you may be miserably seasick even in calm weather, in which case it might be worthwhile talking to your GP about travel-sickness tablets (especially as being seasick could affect the efficacy of your antiepileptic drugs). If you cannot discover a cause and work out a solution for it, then you may have to look at other ways of getting to your destination, such as flying or using the Channel Tunnel.

Can flying in an aeroplane bring on a seizure?

For 99% of people with epilepsy it is safe to travel by aeroplane, but a very small number have reported having a seizure during a flight. There is evidence that low atmospheric pressure at very high altitude can make some people's seizures worse but, as the air pressure in an aeroplane is kept constant, there is no logical reason (except perhaps stress) why anyone's epilepsy should be worse when flying.

If you are planning a very long flight which involves crossing time zones, you will need to remember that this will affect the timing of your medication. It is advisable to adjust the routine gradually over a period of a few days (this also applies to adjusting sleep patterns) rather than make any sudden changes.

I have epilepsy and also use a wheelchair. Will airlines be able to accommodate me?

Airlines claim to have a positive attitude to people with special needs, but in practice this is not always obvious. Good planning should help you avoid any potential problems. Make sure that the airline knows well in advance about your wheelchair, and also about your epilepsy if you still have frequent seizures. They can then arrange for special lifts into the aircraft and allow space so that your access to seating is clear.

Activities and facilities

We are taking our family to a theme park, but because I have epilepsy I am frightened to go on some of the rides with my sons. Should I go on them?

You will almost certainly be asked to join in on rides! The crucial issues are your type of seizure and their frequency. You have to try and work out the chances of a seizure occurring when you are on a ride and how dangerous this might be – this will depend on the nature of the ride, the seizure type and whether your seizures are predictable.

It may help your planning if you can find out full details of the rides before you go. For example, some of these attractions state specifically that people with epilepsy should not use them because they include a flashing light source. Unless you are photosensitive (this is discussed in the section on *More about seizures* in Chapter 1), this should not be a problem. If you cannot get hold of this information, you will have to agree to make the final decision on each individual ride when you get there.

Swimming pools in hotels and on camp sites often do not have lifeguards. Is it safe for me to swim?

If you are a competent swimmer (see *Sports* in Chapter 9), it would be safe to swim provided that you always have someone near to help you should you have a seizure. This 'someone' could be a friend, relative or partner. You should not swim alone and, if the person with you is not a qualified lifesaver, then you should keep to shallower water – it should not be deeper than the accompanying person's shoulder height.

Remember that swimming in open water (rivers, lakes or the sea) is more dangerous than in a swimming pool, and so extra precautions should be taken if you decide to swim in these situations.

We enjoy beach holidays and have usually gone somewhere hot and sunny. This will be our first proper holiday since we were told two years ago that my husband David has epilepsy. Will the heat make his epilepsy worse?

Heat rarely makes epilepsy worse but, if this is true in David's case, then you will probably be aware of it already from your experiences here. If there is no evidence that heat affects his epilepsy before you go, then it is unlikely to be affected by the sun while you are away. Remember that too much exposure to the sun is unsafe for other reasons unconnected with epilepsy – it can increase the risk of skin cancer, especially if you get sunburnt. Like any other adult, your husband should wear a high protection factor suncream and keep out of the sun during the hottest part of the day.

Are there hotels that specialize in providing facilities for people like my wife, who has other medical conditions as well as epilepsy?

There are two national organizations that can provide you with information and advice about holidays for people with special needs like your wife, including lists of suitable hotels. They are the Holiday Care Service and RADAR (Royal Association for Disability and Rehabilitation), and their addresses are in Appendix 1.

I leave school this summer and before I go to college in the autumn I want to travel around Europe with my friends. They are planning to take advantage of those cheap rail tickets for young people and to stay in youth hostels or similar accommodation. Will I be able to stop my parents worrying?

Many young people go on this type of trip these days, and all their parents worry about them. After all, it is often the first time that their children have been away from home and unreachable for any length of time. Your concerns for your parents are very under-standable, and perhaps the best way to deal with them is to reassure yourself that you have planned for any possible problems before you set off and to convince your parents of the same. Your choice of transport and accommodation should not cause you any problems, and it should prove to be an exciting and educational experience.

The two essentials are that you have the correct supplies of medication and the correct travel insurance (both considered in more detail in the next section of this chapter). Check that your friends are confident that they can manage any seizures, should any occur. A copy of the *Epilepsy Passport* (published by the International Bureau for Epilepsy) might be useful for all of them.

Tell your parents that you will ring home regularly to let them know how things are going, and where you are going and when – but as the essence of this type of holiday is its flexibility, they must

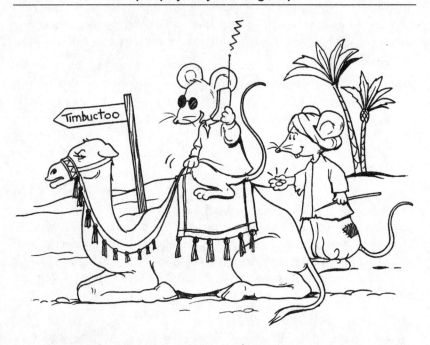

not be surprised if they get a call on a different day from a different country!

Medical care abroad

Will our travel insurance cover epilepsy?

You should check this before you leave for your holiday, as it is important that you have proper insurance in case you need medical help while you are away. It is essential that you give details of your epilepsy and any other existing medical conditions on the insurance application form – they are regarded as 'pre-existing conditions' and, if you do not mention them, they will not be covered. If you have any problems getting travel insurance, then contact the British Epilepsy Association (address in Appendix 1), as this is one of the many types of insurance available through their insurance brokers.

We want to go on holiday abroad, but are unsure about emergency medical facilities. Where can we find out more?

From a number of sources – the holiday company, your travel agent, or the British Embassy in the particular country that you wish to visit. Any addresses you need should be widely available, perhaps in the tour brochure or from your travel agent. The Department of Health produce a leaflet called the *Traveller's guide to health* which you may find useful, and details of how to obtain a copy are in Appendix 2. Once you have the information about your destination, then you will be able to make a sensible decision and, we hope, enjoy an excellent family holiday.

Remember that whatever the level of care available, in many countries you will have to pay some, if not all, of the cost of medical treatment. This means that travel insurance is essential, whether you buy it through your travel agent, your insurance broker or the British Epilepsy Association. Medical attention is free in all European Union countries provided that you have obtained certificate number E111 (from your local Department of Health and Social Security office or Post Office) before you go.

Will my tablets be available abroad if I need a new supply?

Probably, but it depends where you are going. All the major antiepileptic drugs are available in economically developed parts of the world, such as western Europe, the United States and Canada, Australia and New Zealand, and Japan. Their availability elsewhere is much less certain. If you are taking one of the newer drugs such as vigabatrin (Sabril), lamotrigine (Lamictal), gabapentin (Neurontin), topiramate (Topamax) or tiagabine (Gabatril), then you have the additional problem that these drugs are so far only licensed for sale in a small number of countries.

You should also be aware that your tablets may have a different name in another country. The generic name (the true or scientific name of the drug) will be the same but the brand or trade name (the name given to it by the pharmaceutical company that makes it) may not. You can check the names in Table 3.1 or contact the relevant pharmaceutical company or call the British Epilepsy Association helpline (phone number in Appendix 1) where they keep a list of the relevant names. At the same time you could ask about the drug's availability at your destination.

If you add on to all this the fact that you will almost certainly have to pay for any drugs you buy abroad (and they can be very expensive), you will see that it is worth taking a good supply of your tablets with you. In an attempt to avoid any potential problems, it is worth dividing them into two separate packages, keeping one on your person and the other in your hand luggage: suitcases have been known to go astray!

A letter from your doctor stating exactly what has been prescribed for you and why could also be useful, either in case you do need to buy extra supplies or to prevent any difficulties as you go through customs. This letter (which should include the doctor's name and address) may also be of help if a doctor in a foreign country needs more detailed medical information about your epilepsy and its treatment.

You can also obtain an *Epilepsy Passport* through the International Bureau for Epilepsy: this not only lists the various European and American trade names of the major antiepileptic drugs, but also has information about epilepsy in several different European languages and a mini-phrase book.

9
Your social life

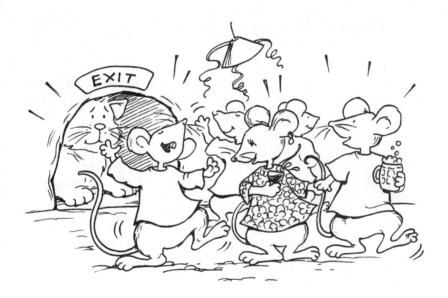

Introduction

In this chapter we concentrate on those activities that you may choose to do, and then on activities which involve flashing or flickering light. The possible links between disco lighting, computer games, television and epilepsy have received publicity that is out of all proportion to the small scale of the problem that

There is a glossary at the end of this book to help you with unfamiliar medical terms.

actually exists. You only need to be concerned if you are photo-sensitive (this is discussed in more detail in the section on *More about seizures* in Chapter 1) and even then there are ways of preventing problems before they occur.

Sports

We're always being told that exercise is good for us. Is that true for people with epilepsy?

Without question exercise is good for people and many really do not exercise enough. This is also the case for people with epilepsy. There is evidence that would suggest that seizures are less likely to occur when someone is active, so exercise could be very beneficial for some people.

However, there is also evidence that some people do tend to have seizures when relaxing after exercise, perhaps whilst showering and changing, so this needs to be kept in mind. Nevertheless, it should not put anyone off taking exercise.

Are there any forms of exercise or sport I should avoid?

Except for some dangerous sports, the vast majority of decisions concerning participation will be based on general safety, not just the activity itself. It is important to consider the inherent dangers in any physical activity, the standard safety measures for every-one, the predictability of your seizures and any supervision, if required. If you are happy with all these factors there are very few activities you should not take part in.

You will need to take all the normal safety precautions required for a particular sport, and then perhaps one or two extra (some of these are discussed in the answers to other questions in this section). However, there are a few less common and higher-risk sports where loss of control due to a seizure could be dangerous, even in the best-supervised circumstances: those that spring to mind are scuba diving and motor sports.

The local swimming club won't let me join. Do you think this is fair?

No. In a controlled environment like a swimming club, swimming for people with epilepsy is perfectly safe, provided that a few commonsense precautions are taken. If you can explain these to the club, then perhaps they will change their minds about allowing you to join.

You should not swim without telling a lifeguard, even if your epilepsy is well controlled. If you have frequent seizures, then it is sensible to go to the club with someone who knows about your epilepsy and is able to take care of you if a seizure occurs.

If you are a non-swimmer, it is very important that you should be able to swim: you are more likely to drown through being a non-swimmer than by having a seizure in a swimming pool supervised by lifeguards. In this case it is even more important that the club lets you join.

If you are a non-swimmer and no qualified lifeguard is available, then you will have to keep to the shallower end of the pool and only swim in water that is no deeper than the shoulder height of a companion you have taken with you.

I am worried about my husband playing rugby – what if he bangs his head?

Any game of rugby is potentially dangerous, but even so thousands of people enjoy the game every weekend. Unless your husband's epilepsy was caused by a bad head injury, it should be possible and safe, within the regulations of the game, for him to take part. There are specific regulations about the protective equipment that may be worn but, if you are particularly concerned, he will probably be allowed to wear a skull cap to protect his head (head collisions are not completely avoidable, even in touch rugby). Perhaps he could talk this through with the club he plays for.

I am anxious about riding a bike. Will it be safe?

It is dangerous for anybody – with or without epilepsy – to cycle in busy traffic, and caution is required even on less busy side roads.

Everybody should wear protective helmets and brightly coloured clothing when they are out on their bikes.

If possible, the best place for you to ride is somewhere where there are specific bike lanes. If you still have unpredictable seizures, then it would be preferable for you to keep to areas where traffic is restricted.

My company are sending everyone in my department on an outdoor pursuits course. Should I go?

Probably. As with other aspects of sport and safety, you must consider the activity to be undertaken, your seizures and the supervision available. The only reason you should not take part is if the activity is inherently dangerous, or your seizures are unpredictable or the relevant supervision and safety equipment cannot be provided. The chances of all this occurring are quite small.

Are your seizures predictable, i.e. are they controlled by medication, have a particular pattern (nocturnal, only on awakening etc.), have an aura or specific 'trigger'? If so, this will help a great deal.

We suppose that the other factor is: do you really want to go? These courses do split opinions on their usefulness.

Night clubs

My friend Sean wants to go a local disco, but someone has told us that they can cause problems for people with epilepsy. What should we do?

There is a lot of incorrect information around on the subject of discos and epilepsy, and it often leads to unnecessary restrictions being placed on people. There is only one reason why Sean should not go to the disco and enjoy himself, and that is if he is photosensitive (discussed in more detail in the section on *More about seizures* in Chapter 1) *and* strobe lighting is to be used. Even if he is photosensitive he would still be safe provided that there were no strobe lights. He could check on the types of lights to be used.

If a strobe light should be unexpectedly switched on, then Sean could reduce its effects by covering one eye with his hand. Closing one eye will not be enough, as light can pass through closed eyelids. This can also be a useful technique for photosensitive people in other situations where flickering lights might cause them problems.

But won't the noise at the night club cause problems?

Loud noise, usually heard without warning, can bring on a seizure in an extremely small number of people. Unless there is already evidence of this in Sean's case, then the noise at the night club will not be a problem.

I went to a party the other night and got rather drunk. I then had a seizure. Does alcohol effect epilepsy and, if so, will I have to stop drinking it completely?

Alcohol is in fact a drug and therefore anyone who drinks it may be affected by it. It can make antiepileptic medication less effective and may actually cause seizures if too much is drunk at one time, although an occasional drink is unlikely to be harmful.

Because drinking alcohol is seen as a symbol of sociability, it is important to find your own level and to avoid drinking too much. You will probably not have to stop drinking alcohol completely, but you will need to get the balance right – this will not only involve thinking about the amount that you drink, but also about sleeping (particularly important) and eating patterns. Both the latter are easily disrupted by too much alcohol.

As medical research suggests that drinking more than two units of alcohol increases the risk of seizures in people with epilepsy, a sensible daily limit would appear to be about one or at most two units. A unit of alcohol is equivalent to one glass of wine *or* half a pint of average strength beer or lager *or* one single measure of spirits. Saving up a daily alcohol 'allowance' for a weekend binge, i.e. drinking 7–14 units over the weekend, would be a mistake and would almost certainly increase the risk of you having a seizure.

Television

The doctor has told me to make sure I do not go close to our TV screen. Why?

It sounds as if you are photosensitive (discussed in more detail in the section on *More about seizures* in Chapter 1), which means that watching television might cause you to have a seizure. The closer you get to the television, the greater the risk, because the screen with its flickering light will fill more of your field of vision. The flicker is caused by the way television works – the picture is recreated on the screen many times a second.

Your doctor's advice is sensible, but this does not mean that you need to stop watching television. With a few sensible precautions you are unlikely to have any additional seizures.

As a rough rule of thumb, you should watch from a distance that is at least four times the size of the screen, i.e. from at least 2 metres (6–7 feet) for a 48–51 cm (20–21 inches) screen, or from at least 2.5 metres (8–9 feet) for a 59 cm (25 inch) model. You should also use a remote control to turn the TV on and off and to change channels.

Turning the brightness control down a little might help, and you may also need to experiment with the lighting in the room where the television is. Some photosensitive people do better watching in a darkened room, while for most others it is better if the room is well lit.

Is it true that small television screens are better than large ones for people with epilepsy?

Yes, but it only applies to those who are photosensitive. It is usually safer for photosensitive people to watch a small screen, about 40 cm (14 inches) across or smaller, as opposed to anything larger. This is about the size of a small portable television. If you want to check the size of your own set, remember that screen size is measured on the diagonal. They should still be watched from a suitable distance, as described in the previous question (for an average small portable this will mean from about 1.5 metres (5 feet) away).

I've heard that wearing sunglasses can help photosensitive people when they are watching television. Does it matter what type of sunglasses they wear?

Sunglasses will not help very much: they will reduce the glare from the screen, but will have no effect on the flicker.

People who are photosensitive can reduce the flicker by covering one eye with their hand or an eye patch. However, this may be inconvenient and it may be better simply to watch TV from at least 2 metres away, preferably a set with a small screen.

Will they ever make televisions that don't affect photosensitive people?

Yes, and in fact they already do. Some televisions now scan the screen at a very fast rate, one which is too fast for the eye to recognize. These 100 Hz televisions are not known to have caused any seizures. You can also buy very small portable televisions which use liquid crystal display (LCD) screens, and these do not flicker at all.

Does watching TV for long periods at a time make epilepsy worse?

It is unlikely to make epilepsy worse unless you are photosensitive or excessively tired. Whether it is good for general well-being to turn yourself into a couch potato is a question we will leave to others to answer! Are you watching TV because you want to and not because you lack confidence about going out (see *Coming to terms with epilepsy* in Chapter 5)?

Computers and computer games

I have been diagnosed as photosensitive and watching TV can be problem. Will using a computer have the same effect?

We all tend to assume that computer monitors and televisions work in the same way – after all, the screen is the same shape and they can both show pictures! However, this is not the case. One of the differences (to be technical for a moment) is that computer monitors flash at a significantly different rate from television screens and also rarely flash at a rate that the human eye can recognize. For example, IBM-compatible machines usually have a flash (reflex) rate of 60 or over per second, a rate which affects very few people, even if they are photosensitive. Most televisions work at a slower rate, and although this is still too rapid for us to be really aware of the flicker, our eyes can still respond to it.

All this simply means that you are unlikely to be affected by using a computer, provided that you use a proper monitor. If a television is being used as the screen for the computer, then that is a different matter and inadvisable, as it could cause some problems. If you are still concerned, then you could consider a computer with a liquid crystal display (LCD) screen which does not flash at all. LCDs are usually found on portable computers, which unfortunately tend to cost considerably more than a desktop model of equivalent power.

Would the filters that you get to fit onto computer screens be of any use?

The filters that you can buy from most computer accessory stores will reduce the glare from the screen, but used alone they have no effect on screen flicker.

10
Relationships, sex and pregnancy

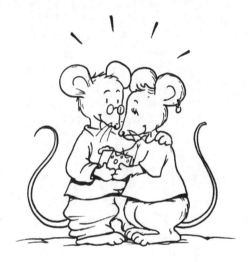

Introduction

There is often a great deal of misinformation provided about relationships, marriage and having a family for people with epilepsy. There is usually no reason why people cannot enjoy the same friendships and family developments as all others. A little more planning is sometimes needed, but this should not prevent

There is a glossary at the end of this book to help you with unfamiliar medical terms.

people doing what they choose. People need to be wary of advice that says no, as it may well be out-of-date.

Relationships

Should I tell my girlfriend about my epilepsy?

Ideally relationships should be built on trust and honesty. It is possible to keep secrets in a close relationship, but it usually imposes a considerable strain on the people involved. If you do not discuss your epilepsy with your girlfriend and she suspects that you are keeping secrets from her, then she may feel that you do not trust her or she may begin to doubt your honesty. There is also the possibility that other people who know about your epilepsy may accidentally or deliberately let the cat out of the bag.

We therefore think that it is a good policy to talk about epilepsy at a fairly early stage in a relationship. This does not mean blurting out the information before asking for a first date! We hope that you have enough confidence in yourself to be able to discuss epilepsy easily, although we appreciate that it is easier for us to say that than for you to do it. It is important to explain to her exactly what your seizures consist of as many people have misconceptions about epilepsy. If your girlfriend is truly looking for a serious relationship with you, then revealing that you have epilepsy should not be a great problem. If she is not, then she may make your epilepsy a convenient excuse for breaking things off – in which case be assured that your epilepsy was not the problem, and that she would have sooner or later found some other reason for ending the relationship.

I sometimes think that nobody will love me or want to marry me because of my epilepsy. What should I do?

Many people with epilepsy enjoy long and happy marriages or other long-term relationships. Having said that, some research studies have suggested that people with epilepsy are less likely to get married than other people, so your fears are not entirely unfounded. We do know that people who are confident enough to talk about their epilepsy positively and in context are more successful at developing relationships than those who do not. We hope that the major theme that has been running through this book is the answer: get to know as much about your epilepsy and yourself as possible, so that you can communicate about it with confidence.

From your question it sounds as if you are still thinking negatively about your epilepsy. Whatever the cause of your lack of self-assurance, the best thing that you can do is to try and change your attitude and be positive about your epilepsy and confident about yourself.

Is there any law that will stop me getting married?

Not in this country. However, this is not true of every country in the world, so if you are considering getting married abroad, then check first with the relevant embassy.

I do not want to tell my potential in-laws about my epilepsy. Is this sensible?

It is understandable that you may be apprehensive about this, especially if you do not know them too well. In our opinion you should tell them, preferably when you feel sufficiently comfortable with them to do so. There are some suggestions about how to tell people about epilepsy in the section on *Outside the family* in Chapter 5. We hope that the reaction that you get will be positive but, if it is not, then you and your boyfriend will have to work together to educate and reassure his parents, and so in time persuade them to change their attitude.

Sex and contraception

Will I be able to have normal sexual relationships? Wouldn't sex start up my seizures again?

Yes, you should be able to have sexual relationships that are as 'normal' as anyone else's and no, sex does not trigger seizures. However, in a very few cases, antiepileptic drugs and/or repeated seizures can reduce someone's interest in sex, and then a doctor should be consulted for advice.

You do not say if you have other medical problems as well as epilepsy. If you do, and you are concerned about how multiple difficulties might affect your sexuality, then we suggest that you get help and advice from an organization called SPOD (Association to aid the Sexual and Personal Relationships of People with a Disability). The address is in Appendix 1.

Will I be able to take the contraceptive pill?

Yes. The efficacy of the contraceptive pill is reduced by some of the major antiepileptic drugs, for example phenytoin (Epanutin) and carbamazepine (Tegretol, Tegretol Retard). This means that a higher-dose pill is needed to provide the same contraceptive effect and efficacy cannot be guaranteed. Other antiepileptic drugs have no affect at all on the pill: examples are sodium valproate (Epilim, Epilim Chrono) and the newer drugs such as vigabatrin (Sabril), lamotrigine (Lamictal), gabapentin (Neurontin) and tiagabine (Gabatril).

Most GP practices now have a staff member, either a doctor or a practice nurse, who specializes in providing advice on contraception, and we would suggest that you talk through all the options with them. After all, you might decide that the pill is not for you for reasons totally unconnected with your epilepsy. If you would prefer not to go to the practice about contraception, then you could go to a family planning clinic, but remember to tell them about your epilepsy and medication.

Pregnancy

Will I be able to get pregnant if I have epilepsy?

There is no reason why you cannot get pregnant. Some studies have suggested that fertility might be slightly reduced in women with epilepsy and some women do indeed find it difficult to become pregnant with epilepsy. This is due to the seizures upsetting the hormonal control of fertility – seizures can alter the

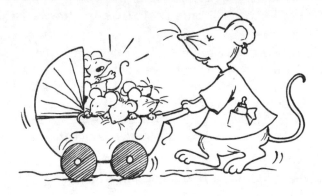

hormones produced during a menstrual cycle. There have been reports that if a woman takes sodium valproate during childhood, she can develop a problem with multiple cysts on her ovaries, where the eggs are produced. If this happens, it can be corrected by a change of antiepileptic therapy. If a woman with epilepsy has not got pregnant after a year of trying, she should go and talk to her doctor about the problem. You may get referred to a specialist fertility clinic.

Do epilepsy drugs cause impotence?

If impotence happens for the first time soon after beginning epilepsy treatment, the problem may be the result of the drug. However, psychological factors also can be very important. If impotence occurs, it is important to go and discuss the problem with your doctor. Some studies have reported a decrease in sexual drive in people who have been on treatment for epilepsy since childhood.

Will it be possible to have a baby while I am on antiepileptic medication?

The answer is yes, and the great majority (about 94%) of women with epilepsy have normal pregnancies and healthy babies. However, there is a risk that the drugs may affect the baby, and we discuss this further in the answer to the next question.

I want to have a baby. Should I talk to my doctor before I get pregnant?

Yes. Preconception counselling for those with epilepsy is very important. In the last few years, there have been many advances in epilepsy treatment; therefore, if there is a local specialist running a preconception clinic, you should ask your GP for a referral. Otherwise, a neurologist or another doctor specializing in epilepsy should be able to answer your questions. Issues that may be discussed will include:

- whether you still need treatment and which is the best treatment;
- taking folate therapy before getting pregnant and for the first three months once you are pregnant;
- seizure control during pregnancy;
- breastfeeding;
- caring for your new baby.

Is antiepileptic medicine dangerous for the unborn baby?

It can be. None of the antiepileptic drugs can be considered 100% safe in pregnancy, although some are safer than others. The newer drugs such as lamotrigine (Lamictal), gabapentin (Neurontin) and possibly tiagabine (Gabatril) look safe, but have not yet been in use for long enough for us to be totally sure. It is important to put this risk into context, as the chances of the baby being affected are only slightly higher than average, and most problems caused are minor and can be corrected once the baby is born. However, some drugs in some women will cause more severe harm to some babies, but such problems are rare.

The most dangerous time for the baby is in the first 12 weeks of pregnancy, which is why doctors advise women with epilepsy to get expert advice and to plan their pregnancies well in advance, so that their treatment can be adjusted if necessary – adjusting or withdrawing treatment can take several weeks or even months.

Is it very serious to have a seizure during pregnancy?

It is very rare for a seizure to cause harm to the unborn baby, but it is advisable to try and keep them to a minimum.

I have epilepsy – will my child have epilepsy?

It is very unlikely, but is does depend on your kind of epilepsy. If your epilepsy is focal or partial, i.e. arises in one part of the brain, the risk is negligible (about one in 20 cases). If you have or have had primary generalized epilepsy, such as absence seizures, the risk is slightly greater (about one in 10). If many people in your family have epilepsy, then the specialist would take a history and be able to give you a clearer indication of the risk of your child developing epilepsy. Types of seizures and epilepsy are covered in more detail in Chapter 1.

You mentioned folate therapy earlier. What dose should I be taking?

It is recommended that all women should take folic acid (0.5 mg/day) for a month before they become pregnant and for the first three months of pregnancy, to try and prevent spina bifida occurring in the new baby. It has been suggested that women with epilepsy should take a slightly higher dose of folic acid (4.0 mg/day) as some of the drugs for epilepsy, particularly sodium valproate and carbamazepine, increase the risk of spina bifida. Both doses of folic acid can be purchased from the chemist without a prescription.

I am very worried that I might have a seizure during labour. Is this likely?

It is unlikely that you will have a seizure during labour. However, if you do have frequent seizures normally and you are worried about the possibility, drugs such as clobazam (Frisium) may be of benefit. This is an antiepileptic drug often used intermittently and in special circumstances. You need to discuss this with your consultant.

I am taking drugs for epilepsy. Can I breastfeed my baby daughter?

There is usually no reason why you cannot breastfeed, although many myths are around. Your baby has been exposed to the drugs that you take for epilepsy while she was in your womb for nine months, and breastfeeding is, in fact, a natural way of weaning the baby off the drugs. Phenobarbitone, benzodiazepines (diazepam, clonazepam) and possibly lamotrigine can make the baby drowsy; if this is a problem, it needs to be discussed with your GP or midwife.

I am worried that I might drop my baby during a seizure whilst I am feeding him. What should I do?

It is suggested that women who have frequent seizures should carry their child as little as possible when feeding. The best option is to feed your child whilst sitting on the floor. The same goes for while you are bathing your baby. It is also a good idea to put cold water in the bath first, so that, if you do have a seizure, there is no risk of burning your baby. Also, use only an inch or so of water. If your seizures are frequent, it would be sensible not to bath your baby unless there is someone else around who can help if necessary.

Periods and HRT

My seizures tend to occur during the time of my period. Why does this happen?

This is quite a common problem. It is called *catamenial epilepsy*. This just means 'around the time of a period'. It is due to your hormone levels changing. Progesterone, the hormone which occurs in the last two weeks of the menstrual cycle, has some protective effects against seizures. Just before the onset of your period, your progesterone levels drop and the protective effect is lost. This may be the reason why you tend to have seizures at this time.

I am approaching the 'change'. What will happen to my epilepsy?

It is difficult to know the exact answer to this question. Some women's epilepsy undoubtedly improves during this time, but for others it does not, and we cannot predict who will improve and who will not. Women, whose seizures tend to cluster around their periods, may find that their seizures become less predictable, occurring at any time.

Can I take hormone replacement therapy?

There is very little information about hormone replacement therapy and epilepsy. However, many of the drugs used to treat epilepsy do make the bones thinner than normal. We suggest that it is certainly worth your doctor trying you on various preparations to see if one will suit you.

Glossary

absence seizures Generalized seizures involving a brief loss of awareness for several (perhaps 5–20) seconds. They usually occur many times a day, every day, and are often accompanied by eyelid fluttering or lip-smacking or chewing movements.

acupuncture A complementary therapy in this country but a traditional form of treatment in China, acupuncture involves inserting special very fine needles into the skin at particular sites on the body in order to balance the 'life energy' or 'vital force' which the Chinese call 'ch'i' or 'qi'.

AED An abbreviation for antiepileptic drug.

akinetic seizures Derived from the Greek and meaning 'without movement or motion', this is an older and less appropriate name for astatic or atonic seizures.

ambulatory monitoring A portable type of EEG – it literally means 'EEG monitoring while walking about' (from the Latin word *ambulare* meaning 'to walk'). It allows brainwaves to be recorded continuously over anything from several hours to a few days, a much longer time period than is possible with a routine EEG in the out-patients department of a hospital.

anticonvulsant drugs Another name for antiepileptic drugs.

antiepileptic drugs Drugs used to treat epilepsy, also known as anticonvulsant drugs or AEDs.

aromatherapy A complementary therapy involving treatment with essential oils, which are aromatic (scented) oils extracted from the roots, flowers or leaves of plants by distillation. Aromatherapy often involves massage, but the oils can also be inhaled or added to baths.

astatic seizures Another name for atonic seizures.

ataxia Jerky, clumsy, uncoordinated movements.

atonic seizures Generalized seizures involving sudden loss of muscle tone, i.e. sudden relaxation of the muscles, resulting in a fall. An atonic seizure usually lasts for a few seconds, and may be preceded by a very brief myoclonic seizure. 'Atonic' and 'astatic' both come from the Greek: 'atonic' means 'without tone or strength', while 'astatic' means 'unstable' or 'unable to stand'.

attack Another name for a seizure.

aura A strange sensation, feeling, smell or taste that acts as a warning that a seizure is about to happen. The word 'aura' comes from the Latin and literally means 'breeze'. Not everyone experiences an aura as part of a seizure – people who do usually have tonic-clonic seizures or complex partial seizures which start in either the temporal lobe or the frontal lobe. An aura is actually a brief simple partial sensory seizure.

autism Autistic people are unable to respond to other people, are extremely resistant to change of any kind, have difficulty learning to talk or to communicate in other ways, and often have additional behavioural problems.

benign Generally speaking, a condition or illness which is not serious and does not usually have harmful consequences. In describing epilepsy it can mean either that the seizures are usually controlled very easily with a single antiepileptic drug, or that the epilepsy usually goes into spontaneous remission by late childhood.

benign rolandic epilepsy of childhood Full name for the abbreviation BREC.

biofeedback A complementary therapy based on the fact that it is easier to learn how to alter some aspect of your physical or mental state, i.e. to develop conscious control of your body's reactions, if you get some sort of reward each time you manage to make the desired change (the 'feedback' part of the name – 'bio' simply means life).

brain scan A painless and completely harmless way of producing clear and detailed pictures of the brain. The two main types are CT scans and MRI; others are PET and SPECT scans.

brainstem The lowest part of the brain, lying right underneath the cerebral hemispheres. It joins all the other parts of the brain to the spinal cord. The brainstem controls breathing and heartbeat, and is involved in the coordination of certain activities including swallowing and eye movements.

brainwaves Common name for the tiny electrical signals produced inside the brain.

brand name or trade name   Most drugs have at least two names: the brand or trade name is the name given to a drug by its manufacturer, and is usually written with a capital first letter. The other name is the generic name.

BREC   This is the commonly-used abbreviation for benign rolandic epilepsy of childhood, a common epilepsy syndrome in children. It usually starts at between 4 and 9 years of age and all children grow out of it by their teenage years. Most of the seizures are simple partial seizures involving the face and neck. These seizures may then become secondary generalized tonic-clonic seizures. The EEG usually shows a character-istic pattern. Some children do not require treatment with an anti-epileptic drug because the seizures may be very infrequent. Seizure control is good or excellent in those children who are prescribed anti-epileptic drugs.

catamenial seizures   Seizures which are caused or made worse by menstruation (periods) are called catamenial seizures (from the Greek word *katamenios* which means monthly).

CAT scan   Another name for a CT scan.

cerebellum   A part of the brain lying just under the back of the two cerebral hemispheres. It is connected to many other areas of the brain and to the spinal cord. The cerebellum is involved with the control of movements, and coordinates the action of all the different muscles.

cerebral hemispheres   The two halves of the cerebrum. Each hemi-sphere consists of four areas called lobes. The hemispheres are involved in most of our conscious activities and ways of behaving. The left hemisphere controls everything that happens down the right-hand side of the body, while the right hemisphere controls what happens down the left-hand side.

cerebral palsy   A medical condition caused by damage to the brain before, during or soon after birth. People with cerebral palsy have pro-blems and difficulties with movement, posture and muscle function, and with weakness of the limbs. 'Cerebral' comes from the Latin word *cerebrum* meaning 'brain', and 'palsy' is another word for 'paralysis' meaning 'loss of movement or motion'.

cerebrum   The largest part of the brain, divided into halves called cerebral hemispheres.

classification   Generally speaking, to group related topics together into categories in an organized and logical way. In epilepsy, seizures, syndromes and types of epilepsy are classified by where they start in the brain, what is known about their causes, the effects they have, and so on.

There is an internationally-agreed system for this, and by following it doctors can ensure that they all know exactly which type of epilepsy is being described. Knowing the correct epilepsy classification also helps doctors to decide on the most suitable treatment.

clinical diagnosis The identification of an illness or medical disorder based on what the doctor observes and is told about the symptoms.

clonic seizures Generalized seizures involving repeated and rhythmic contractions of the muscles, causing jerks or twitches of the limbs or the whole body. They usually last for between 30 seconds and 1–2 minutes but sometimes last longer. 'Clonic' comes from the Greek word *klonos*, meaning 'turmoil'.

community care assessment The way in which professional staff from a Social Services department work out which community care services someone needs. Community care services are intended to support people who need help with daily living, perhaps because of long-term illness, and enable them to live as full and independent lives as possible, often in their own homes. The amount of care provided will depend on what is needed and on the resources which are available locally.

complementary therapies Non-medical treatments which may be used in addition to conventional medical treatments. Popular complementary therapies include acupuncture, aromatherapy and homeopathy. Some of these therapies are available through the NHS, but this is unusual, and depends on individual hospitals and GPs.

complex partial seizures Partial seizures during which someone's level of consciousness or awareness is affected – the person having the seizure may lose consciousness, or look confused or dazed, or behave in a strange way.

compliance Following medical advice correctly or taking treatment exactly as prescribed. Research has shown that people who are well-informed about their treatment and the reasons for it are more likely to comply with it than those who have not been given the full details.

computed tomography or computerized tomography/computer assisted tomography/computerized axial tomography Alternative names for a CT scan.

convulsion Another name for a seizure.

convulsive status epilepticus Status epilepticus arising from tonic-clonic seizures.

corpus callosum The band of nerve fibres joining the two cerebral hemispheres together.

cryptogenic epilepsy   Describes epilepsy where a cause is suspected but none can actually be found.

CT scan   A type of brain scan which uses X-rays to produce images of the brain which are then fed into a computer. The computer reconstructs these images into 'slices' – pictures of cross-sections of the brain. When these pictures are viewed in the correct order, they build up a picture of the whole brain. CT stands for computed or computerized tomography (tomography comes from two Greek words – *tomos* meaning 'a slice' and *graphein* meaning 'to draw'). It is also referred to as CAT scanning (computer assisted tomography or computerized axial tomography).

cyanosis   When the skin turns a blue colour because there is not enough oxygen in the blood. It comes from the Greek word *kyanos* which means 'blue'.

déjà vu   A French phrase which means 'already seen', this is the 'I've been here before' feeling.

developmental delay   When a child's physical, mental, emotional and social skills are not developing as they should.

discharges   Out-of-the-ordinary brainwave patterns that appear on an EEG recording. They show that the electrical signals in the brain are not being sent smoothly and in the correct order. The shapes of the discharges and how frequently they occur during the recording provide information about the seizure type.

dominant hemisphere   Although both cerebral hemispheres are important, one usually does far more work than the other. Whichever does the most work is called the dominant hemisphere. In right-handed people (most of the population), the left hemisphere is dominant; in left-handed people, the right hemisphere is usually the dominant one. The control of speech and language usually lies within the dominant hemisphere.

drop attacks or drop seizures   Older names for atonic or astatic seizures.

EEG   An EEG is a completely safe and painless test which records and measures the tiny electrical signals produced inside the brain. It provides a picture of the electrical activity inside the brain, whether it be the normal activity that goes on all the time or the 'out of the correct order' activity that occurs during a seizure. An EEG recording consists of several lines, and each line is a picture of the electrical activity in a different part of the brain (determined by the placing of the electrodes). This means that the EEG can show not only what is happening, but also where in the brain it is happening. EEGs are invaluable tools in the investigation and classification of epilepsy, although they are not a substitute for a clinical diagnosis. They are used to support a clinical diagnosis of epilepsy, and to help decide what type of seizure is involved.

efficacy The ability to produce an intended result. A description usually applied to drugs and how well they work.

electrodes Small discs placed on a person's head during an EEG recording to pick up the brainwaves and transfer them to the EEG machine.

encephalitis An infection causing inflammation (swelling) of the brain.

excitatory neurotransmitters Types of neurotransmitters which work to cause messages to be sent from one neuron to another. They are called excitatory neurotransmitters because they excite or stimulate the neurons.

eyewitness The person who actually sees someone having a seizure. Before a diagnosis can be made, a doctor needs to be given a very clear, detailed and accurate account of precisely what happened just before, during and after a seizure. The eyewitness is the person who can provide this very important information.

febrile convulsions or febrile seizures Convulsions caused by a high temperature (fever). They tend to occur in young children during a feverish illness, but are unlikely after a child is 4 years old. Febrile seizures are *not* epilepsy.

fit Another name for a seizure.

focal seizures Another name for simple partial seizures or complex partial seizures.

frontal lobes The areas of the cerebral hemispheres involved in the control of our voluntary movements and some aspects of our behaviour and emotions.

generalized seizures These occur when the abnormal electrical activity that causes a seizure involves both sides of the brain at once, i.e. the vast majority of the brain. Generalized seizures can be further divided into six types: absence seizures; atonic or astatic seizures; clonic seizures; myoclonic seizures; tonic seizures; and tonic-clonic seizures.

generic name Most drugs have at least two names: the generic name is the scientific name (usually written with a small first letter) and applies to all the versions of that drug, regardless of the manufacturer. The other name is the brand name.

genes The 'units' of heredity that determine which characteristics we inherit from our parents.

grand mal　A French phrase which means 'great illness', this is an older name for tonic-clonic seizures.

hemispheres　A shorthand way of referring to the cerebral hemispheres.

history　Information about, and a description of, what actually happened before, during and after a seizure. A full medical history will also include other information about someone's health now and also about what has occurred in the past, perhaps even back as far as when they were born.

homeopathy　A complementary therapy based on the principle that 'like can be cured by like' (the word homeopathy comes from two Greek words that mean 'similar' and 'suffering'). The remedies used contain very dilute amounts of a substance which in larger quantities would produce similar symptoms to the illness being treated. Although there is as yet no scientific evidence for why homeopathy works, it is available through the NHS, although the provision is limited.

hyperventilation　Overbreathing – breathing very much harder, very much faster and far more deeply than normal. People are encouraged to hyperventilate during a routine EEG in order to unmask any abnormal electrical activity in the brain. This technique is particularly useful in diagnosing typical absence seizures.

hypnotherapy　A complementary therapy which uses hypnosis. A person who is hypnotized enters a state of very deep relaxation, during which they are more receptive to suggestions of ways of altering behaviour than they would be in a fully conscious state. Whilst it is most useful in reinforcing good intentions to change bad habits, e.g. stopping smoking, it can also be helpful in reducing stress and increasing confidence.

hypsarrhythmia　A pattern of discharges on an EEG recording. The name comes from the Greek words *hypsi* meaning 'aloft' and *arrhythmos* meaning 'absence of rhythm'. A good translation of hypsarrhythmia is 'mountainous chaos' as the EEG recording is full of jumbled irregular peaks.

ictal　During a seizure. For example, an ictal EEG is one recorded while a seizure is actually taking place. From the Latin word *ictus*, which means a strike or sudden blow – the Latin phrase for an epileptic seizure is *ictus epilepticus*.

idiopathic epilepsy or primary epilepsy　Describes epilepsy for which no obvious cause can be found. 'Idiopathic' means 'of unknown cause' and comes from two Greek words: *idios* meaning 'own' and *pathos* meaning 'suffering'.

incidence   The incidence of a medical condition is the number of people developing it for the first time during each year, i.e. the number of new cases within a year.

infantile spasms   Another name for West syndrome.

inhibitory neurotransmitters   Types of neurotransmitters which work to prevent or stop messages being sent from one neuron to another. They are called inhibitory neurotransmitters because they inhibit or hold back the messages.

interictal   Between seizures. For example, an interictal EEG is one recorded between seizures. *Inter* is a Latin word meaning 'between', and 'ictal' comes from another Latin word *ictus*, which means a strike or sudden blow (the Latin phrase for an epileptic seizure is *ictus epilepticus*).

intramuscular   Into or within a muscle. Often used to describe an injection.

intravenous   Into or within a vein. Often used to describe an injection.

jerk attacks or jerk seizures   Older names for myoclonic seizures.

ketogenic diet   A medically supervised diet which is sometimes tried as a treatment for the more difficult-to-control types of epilepsy. 'Ketogenic' comes from two other words: 'keto' from 'ketones', which are natural substances found in the blood and urine, and formed from the metabolism (breakdown in the body) of fats; and 'genic' meaning to produce or make. Thus the diet is literally one which 'makes lots of ketones'. It consists mainly of fat, is not very tasty, and must be kept to very strictly under the supervision of a hospital dietician.

learning difficulties   Children with learning difficulties have problems in acquiring the practical and behavioural skills needed to cope with everyday living. Learning difficulties can range from the mild, i.e. simply being slower than other children of the same age in developing these skills, to the severe, i.e. being unable to develop enough of these skills ever to allow independent living without considerable daily support from other people.

Lennox–Gastaut syndrome   This is an uncommon epilepsy syndrome which starts at between 1 and 6 years of age. Many different types of seizure may occur, including tonic, atonic, tonic-clonic and myoclonic seizures. Status epilepticus may also occur. There is a characteristic EEG showing a pattern called slow spike and slow wave activity. The seizures in this syndrome are usually resistant to most antiepileptic drugs, and therefore seizure control may be difficult. Children commonly develop moderate or severe learning difficulties and usually require special schooling.

lesion   A general term for any damage or disease affecting a part of the body.

licence   The permit which sets out how, when and for whom a drug should be prescribed.

lobes or lobes of the cerebrum   The areas which make up the two cerebral hemispheres. There are four lobes in each hemisphere: the frontal lobes, the occipital lobes, the parietal lobes and the temporal lobes. Each lobe controls or coordinates specific activities or functions of the body.

magnetic resonance imaging   Full name for the abbreviation MRI.

meningitis   An infection causing inflammation (swelling) of the membranes (layers of tissue) that cover the brain and spinal cord (these membranes are called the meninges).

monotherapy   In epilepsy, the use of only one antiepileptic drug for treatment.

MRI   A type of brain scan which uses magnetism to produce images of the brain which are then fed into a computer. The computer reconstructs these images into pictures of the brain which are similar to those produced by a CT scan but much more detailed. MRI stands for magnetic resonance imaging.

myoclonic seizures   Generalized seizures involving sudden jerky or shock-like contractions of different muscles anywhere in the body, but usually in the arms or legs. Each myoclonic seizure lasts for a fraction of a second, or for one second at most. 'Myoclonic' is derived from the Greek: *myo*- means 'to do with muscles and 'clonic' comes from *klonos*, meaning 'turmoil'.

nausea   Feeling sick, wanting to vomit.

nerve cells   Another name for neurons.

neurologist   A doctor who specializes in treating conditions affecting the brain and nervous system.

neurons   The nerve cells that make up the brain and the nervous system. Neurons are responsible for controlling all the actions and functions of every part of the body – seeing, hearing, talking, walking and even thinking. They are the means by which the brain receives, transmits and interprets messages throughout the body. They work by electricity: tiny electrical signals are sent along the neurons, between the neurons throughout the brain, and then down into the spinal cord where they can be relayed to any of the other nerves in the body. The actual electrical signals or messages are in the form of chemicals called neurotransmitters.

neurotransmitters Chemicals in the brain and nervous system that relay electrical messages between neurons. 'Neuro' means to do with nerve cells and 'transmitters' send or communicate signals or messages. There are many different types of neurotransmitter, including excitatory neurotransmitters and inhibitory neurotransmitters.

night-time seizures Another name for nocturnal seizures.

nocturnal seizures 'Nocturnal' comes from the Latin word *nocturnus* meaning 'during the night'. Because most people sleep at night, this phrase is used to describe seizures that occur during sleep.

non-compliance Refusing, failing or 'forgetting' to follow medical advice or a prescribed course of treatment, e.g. not taking the correct amount of a drug at the correct time of day. The opposite of compliance.

non-convulsive status epilepticus Status epilepticus arising from absence seizures or complex partial seizures.

non-epileptic attacks or non-epileptic seizures Alternative terms for pseudoseizures.

occipital lobes The areas of the cerebral hemispheres involved in vision and our interpretation of what we see.

oral To do with the mouth. For example, oral medication is designed to be taken by mouth and swallowed.

paediatric neurologist A neurologist who concentrates on, and works only with children.

paediatrician A doctor who specializes in treating children.

paraesthesia Pins and needles in the arms or legs.

parietal lobes The areas of the cerebral hemispheres involved in our perception of touch (feeling, and in control of some of our involuntary movements. They are also involved in skills such as reading, writing and dressing.

partial seizures These occur when the abnormal electrical activity that causes a seizure starts in one cerebral hemisphere or in one lobe of one hemisphere. The sensations felt during a partial seizure are determined by the lobe in which the seizure starts. There are two types of partial seizures, called simple partial seizures and complex partial seizures.

perioral cyanosis Cyanosis noticeable around the lips and mouth. *Peri* is a Greek word meaning 'around' or 'near', and 'oral' comes from the Latin and means 'to do with the mouth'.

petit mal   A French phrase which means 'little illness', this is an older name for absence seizures or absence epilepsy.

PET scan   A type of brain scan which provides information about how the brain is functioning as well as showing its structure. At present its use is limited to a few specialized centres. PET stands for positron emission tomography.

photosensitive epilepsy   A reflex epilepsy in which seizures can be brought on by lights flashing or flickering at certain frequencies (numbers of times per second), by strobe lighting, by flickering television sets and other similar triggers. Photosensitivity means being sensitive or susceptible to flashing or flickering lights ('photo-' comes from the Greek and means 'to do with light').

positron emission tomography   Full name for a PET scan.

postictal   After a seizure. For example, the postictal phase describes the time after a seizure. *Post* is a Latin word meaning 'after', and 'ictal' comes from another Latin word *ictus*, which means a strike or sudden blow (the Latin phrase for an epileptic seizure is *ictus epilepticus*).

prevalence   The proportion of a population with a particular medical condition at any one time.

primary epilepsy   Another name for idiopathic epilepsy.

prognosis   A medical assessment of the outlook, expected outcome or probable future course of an illness or disorder.

pseudoseizures or pseudo-epileptic seizures   Seizures which look like epileptic seizures but are not, and which often have an underlying psychological cause. They are more common in girls than in boys, and also in teenagers rather than in younger children. Non-epileptic seizures or attacks is an alternative term for pseudoseizures, and one which is preferred by many doctors.

rectal   To do with the rectum (the back passage, also referred to as the anus).

reflex epilepsies   A rare group of epilepsies in which a seizure can occur in response to a specific trigger or stimulus. The best-known example is photosensitive epilepsy.

repeated jerking attacks or repeated jerking seizures   Older names for clonic seizures.

respite care   Any facility or resource which allows those who care for sick, frail, elderly or disabled relatives or friends to have a break from their caring tasks. Respite care may be provided in residential or nursing homes, in the person's own home, or with another family.

Sapphire nurse An epilepsy specialist nurse provided by the British Epilepsy Association.

scan In this book, a shorthand way of referring to a brain scan.

secondary epilepsy Another name for symptomatic epilepsy.

secondary generalized tonic-clonic seizures or secondarily generalized tonic-clonic seizures Seizures which start as partial seizures but then spread to become generalized seizures involving the vast majority of the brain.

sedation EEG An EEG recording during which anyone who has difficulty lying still is given a sedative to help him or her relax or even go to sleep.

seizures Sudden and uncontrolled episodes of excessive electrical activity in the brain. In epilepsy the fault usually lies in a loss of balance between the different neurotransmitters. When this happens the electrical signals between the neurons are no longer sent smoothly and in the correct order. Instead they are sent out of order, and this 'out of the correct order' signal then often causes an epileptic seizure. This seizure may take the form of a sudden loss of consciousness, involuntary movements, a change in behaviour or a combination of all of these.

side effects Almost all drugs affect the body in ways beyond their intended actions. These unwanted 'extra' effects are called side effects. Side effects vary in their severity from person to person, and sometimes disappear when a body becomes used to a particular drug.

simple partial seizures Partial seizures during which someone's level of consciousness or awareness is not affected: there is no loss of consciousness and the person remains completely aware of what is happening.

simple partial sensory seizures Simple partial seizures which involve a change in sensation such as a strange (often unpleasant) smell or taste, or unexplained fear, or a feeling of déjà vu (the I've been here before' feeling), or even tingling and numbness in the face or an arm. An aura is an example of a simple partial sensory seizure.

single photon emission computerized tomography Full name for a SPECT scan.

sleep-deprived EEG A specialized type of EEG recording. Reducing sleep can cause changes in the electrical signals in the brain (it is rare for it to provoke a seizure). These changes would not be seen in a routine

EEG, but when they appear after sleep deprivation they may provide important evidence to support a diagnosis of epilepsy.

slices   Pictures of cross-sections of the brain produced by a brain scan.

SPECT scan   A type of brain scan which provides information about how the brain is functioning as well as showing its structure. At present its use is limited to a few specialized centres. SPECT stands for single photon emission computerized tomography.

spike and slow wave   A characteristic pattern which often appears in an EEG recording of someone with epilepsy. This pattern is usually seen in children with generalized seizures.

spinal cord   An extension of the brain which runs from the brainstem down the back inside the bones of the spine. The spinal cord relays information between the brain and the rest of the body, and also controls many of our reflexes.

split screen EEG   Another name for videotelemetry.

spontaneous remission   When an illness gets better of its own accord, it is said to have gone into spontaneous remission. In epilepsy, this means that seizures have stopped or 'gone away' and that antiepileptic drugs are no longer needed. However, spontaneous remission only happens in certain types of epilepsy and it is not easy to predict, or even to know exactly when the epilepsy has 'gone away'.

status epilepticus   The currently internationally-accepted definition of status epilepticus is either (a) any seizure lasting for at least 30 minutes or (b) repeated seizures lasting for 30 minutes or longer, from which the person did not regain consciousness between each seizure. Status epilepticus is a Latin phrase which simply means 'in an epileptic condition'. It is always a medical emergency.

stiffening attacks or stiffening seizures   Older names for tonic seizures.

strobe   Abbreviation for either stroboscope or strobe lighting (stroboscope is the name for the equipment used to produce strobe lighting). Strobe lighting uses high-intensity (extremely bright), flashing lights: the number of flashes per second can be altered very precisely to make moving objects appear stationary. They are often used in discos and amusement arcades, and sometimes used to produce special effects in theatres.

symptomatic epilepsy or secondary epilepsy   Describes epilepsy where there is a known cause or for which a cause has been identified.

syndrome A cluster of signs and symptoms occurring together in a non-fortuitous, i.e. non-random or non-coincidental, manner.

telemetry A shorthand way of referring to videotelemetry.

temporal lobe epilepsy Complex partial seizures starting in the temporal lobes of the brain.

temporal lobes The areas of the cerebral hemispheres that control our speech, language and hearing, our feelings of fear and anger, and our bowel and bladder functions. The lobes are also involved in behaviour.

tonic seizures Generalized seizures involving sudden stiffness of the limbs or the whole body, leading to a fall, often like a tree being felled. The seizure usually ends after 5–10 seconds. 'Tonic' comes from the Greek word *tonos*, meaning 'tension'.

tonic-clonic seizures Generalized seizures involving a tonic stage followed by a clonic stage, ie sudden stiffness and a fall followed by repeated and rhythmic muscle contractions. Most tonic-clonic seizures last 1–3 minutes.

trade name Another name for brand name.

tuberous sclerosis An inherited disorder affecting the skin, the nervous system and other organs in the body, which can give rise to epilepsy amongst other symptoms.

tumour An abnormal swelling that forms when cells in a specific area of the body reproduce and increase in number far more quickly than normal.

turn Another name for a seizure.

videotelemetry The literal meaning of 'telemetry' is 'measurement from a distance'. Videotelemetry uses a video camera linked to an EEG machine, and this combination allows simultaneous recording of what a person is doing and his or her brainwaves. When the videotape is played back, one half of the screen shows the person's activities and the other half the EEG recording, and this explains the alternative name for this test – 'split screen EEG'. This means that the clinical evidence (i.e. what is actually happening) and the electrical evidence (the EEG recording) can be looked at together.

West syndrome Also known as infantile spasms, and named after a Dr West who, over 150 years ago, described infantile spasms occurring in his own son. Infantile spasms are a particular type of myoclonic seizure which usually occur in young children between 3 and 10 months old. The spasms usually occur in clusters, with each cluster consisting of 10–50 spasms or more. The spasms are most often seen when the child wakes up and they may be obvious (affecting the whole body, or the arms and legs) or more subtle (affecting only the head or just the eyelids).

Appendix 1
Epilepsy associations and other organizations

National and regional associations

British Epilepsy Association
Anstey House
40 Hanover Square
Leeds LS3 1BE
Tel: 0113 243 9393
Fax: 0113 242 8804
Helpline tel: 0800 309030
Website: http\\:www.epilepsy.org.uk (commended for its layout)

Belfast regional office:
Graham House
Knockbracken Health Care Park
Saintfield Road
Belfast BT8 8BH
Tel: 01232 799355
Fax: 01232 799076
The British Epilepsy Association aims to provide help and support for everyone with epilepsy, their families and those who care for them. This includes helping to provide epilepsy specialist nurses (called Sapphire Nurses) in some areas of the country.

The National Information Centre provides advice and information on any aspect of epilepsy. Enquiries are dealt with by letter or by telephone on the free Epilepsy Helpline. Advice is also available at BEA's regional office in Belfast.

A comprehensive range of literature is available (including a quarterly

magazine called *Epilepsy Today*), as well as many video titles which you
can hire or purchase. Schools' information packs are also available. The
BEA organizes a national network of self-help groups to provide local
contact points for help, information and social events. Among other
services, the BEA can help with all types of insurance through its
brokers.

Epilepsy Association of Scotland
48 Govan Road
Glasgow G51 1JL
Tel: 0141 427 4911
The Epilepsy Association of Scotland provides advice and information,
education/lecturing services, literature, self-help groups and employment training.

Wales Epilepsy Association Cyf
15 Chester Street
St Asaph
Denbighshire LL17 0RE
Tel/Fax: 01745 584444
Helpline: Health Promotion Scheme
Bromfield House
Queen's Lane
Mold
Flintshire
Tel: 0345 413774
The Wales Epilepsy Association provides advice and information, and
has local self-help groups.

Mersey Region Epilepsy Association
The Glaxo Centre
Norton Street
Liverpool L3 8LR
Tel: 0151 298 2666
This is a regional association that provides advice and information, lit-
erature, lectures and a network of self-help groups in Merseyside and
North Wales.

Brainwave – The Irish Epilepsy Association
249 Crumlin Road
Dublin 12
Ireland
Tel: 00 3531 455 7500 (from UK)
email: brainwave@iol.ie
The Irish Epilepsy Association provides for Ireland a similar range of services to those provided by the British Epilepsy Association.

International organizations

International Bureau for Epilepsy
PO Box 21
2100 AA Heemstede
The Netherlands
Tel: 00 3123 5291019
email: ibe@xs40all.nl
The staff (who speak excellent English) will provide details of epilepsy associations throughout the world.

Other epilepsy organizations

The David Lewis Centre
Mill Lane
Warford
Nr Alderly Edge
Cheshire SK9 7UD
Tel: 01565 640000
The David Lewis Centre provides assessment, respite care, and long-term care and education for children and adults with severe epilepsy and learning difficulties.

National Society for Epilepsy
Chalfont Centre for Epilepsy
Chalfont St Peter
Bucks SL9 0RJ
Tel: 01494 601300
website: http://www.erg.ion.ucl.ac.uk/NSEhome

The National Society for Epilepsy provides residential care, respite care and assessment for adults with severe epilepsy and learning difficulties. It has a small network of self-help groups in the community and provides training and training packages for health and other professionals, and advice and information on epilepsy (including a wide ranging set of literature and video packages).

Park Hospital for Children
Old Road
Headington
Oxford OX3 7LQ
Tel: 01865 741717
The Park Hospital for Children provides assessment for children with severe epilepsy, often with associated learning difficulties.

St Elizabeth's School
South End
Much Hadham
Hertfordshire SG10 6EW
Tel: 01279 843451
St Elizabeth's School provides long-term care and education for children with severe epilepsy and learning difficulties.

St Pier's
St Pier's Lane
Lingfield
Surrey RH7 6PW
Tel: 01342 832243
Website: http://www.stpiers.org.uk
St Pier's Lane provides assessment and long-term care and education for children and young adults with severe epilepsy and learning difficulties.

Services for People with Epilepsy
Head Office
Quarrier's Village
Bridge of Weir
Renfrewshire PA11 3SX
Tel: 01505 612224
Services for People with Epilepsy provides assessment and long-term care for adults with epilepsy and learning difficulties.

Other useful organizations

Carers National Association
20-25 Glasshouse Yard
London EC1A 4JS
Tel: 0171 490 8818
Helpline tel: 0171 490 8898 (1.00 pm – 4.00 pm)

CNA in Scotland:
162 Buchanan Street
Glasgow G1 2LL
Tel: 0141 333 9495
email: internet@carersscotland.demon.co.uk
The Carers National Association supports all people who have to care
for others due to medical or other problems.

Continence Foundation
2 Doughty Street
London WC1N 2PH
Tel: 0171 404 6875

Continence Advisory Service Helpline
Tel: 0191 213 0050 (2pm – 7pm weekdays)

DIAL UK
Park Lodge
St Catherine's Hospital
Tickhill Road
Doncaster DN4 8QN
Tel: 0130 231 0123
email: dialuk@aol.com
Website: http://www.members.aol.com/dialuk
DIAL UK gives advice on all aspects of disability.

Disability on the Agenda
FREEPOST
MID 02164
Stratford upon Avon CV37 9BR
Tel: 0345 622 633 (calls charged at local rates)
Textphone: 0345 622 644 (calls charged at local rates)

Disability on the Agenda provides leaflets and up-to-date information on the Disability Discrimination Act.

Disabled Living Foundation
380–384 Harrow Road
London W9 2HU
Tel: 0171 289 6111
Helplines: 0870 603 9177; 0870 603 9176 (for hard-of-hearing)
email: dlfinfo@dlf.org.uk
Website: http://www.dlf.org.uk
Disabled Living Foundation provides information on all kinds of equipment for people with special needs.

DVLA (Driver and Vehicle Licensing Agency)
Drivers' Medical Unit
Longview Road
Morriston
Swansea SA99 1TU
Contact the DVLA for enquiries about driving licences.

Employment Service
National Office
Sanctuary Building
Great Smith Street
London SW1P 3BT
and
Moorfoot
Sheffield S1 4PQ
Tel: 01142 753275
Employment Service provides information on employment advice for people with health problems.

Golden Key
1 Hare Street
Sheerness
Kent ME12 1AH
Tel: 01795 663403
Golden Key sells medical identification bracelets and necklaces.

Headway (National Head Injuries Association Limited)
47 King Edward Court
King Edward Street
Nottingham NG1 1EW
Tel: 0115 924 0800
email: headway@national.demon.co.uk
Website: http://www.national.demon.co.uk
Headway provides support and advice for people who have suffered head injuries.

Health Education Authority (HEA)
Trevelyan House
30 Great Peter Street
London SW1P 2HW
Tel: 0171 222 5300
Website: http://www.hea.org.uk
HEA promotes and provides publications and videos on all aspects of general health, e.g. healthy eating, sensible drinking, stopping smoking, exercise.

Holiday Care Service
2nd Floor
Imperial Buildings
Victoria Road
Horley
Surrey RH6 7PZ
Tel: 0129 377 4535
Holiday Care Service gives holiday advice for people with special needs.

Medic-Alert Foundation
1 Bridge Wharf
156 Caledonian Road
London N1 9UU
Tel: 0171 833 3034
email: info@medicalert.co.uk
Medic-Alert Foundation sells medical identification bracelets and necklaces.

MENCAP
Mencap National Centre
123 Golden Lane
London EC1Y 0RT
Tel: 0171 454 0454
MENCAP provides advice and support for people with learning disabilities, their families and carers through a network of local offices and clubs. Includes the Federation of Gateway Clubs.

National Autistic Society
393 City Road
London EC1V 1NE
Tel: 0171 833 2299
email: nas@nas.org.uk
Website: http://www.oneworld.org/autism_uk
The National Autistic Society provides advice and information on autism for families and professionals. It owns and manages a number of schools and adult communities for people with autism.

National Council for Voluntary Organisations (NCVO)
Regent's Wharf
8 All Saints Street
London N1 9RL
Tel: 0171 713 6161
email: ncvo@compuserve.com
Website: http://www.ncvo/vol.org.uk
The NCVO is the voice of the voluntary sector. Contact for details of any charities in which you may be interested.

Patients Association
18 Guilford Street
London WC1N 1DT
Helpline: 0181 423 8999
The Patients Association provides advice on patients' rights.

RADAR (Royal Association for Disability and Rehabilitation)
12 City Forum
250 City Road
London EC1V 8AF
Tel: 0171 250 3222

RADAR aims to improve the rights and care of disabled people. Information, advice and publications available on topics such as holidays, mobility, leisure, education and employment.

Royal Society for the Prevention of Accidents (RoSPA)
Edgbaston Park
353 Bristol Road
Birmingham B5 7ST
Tel: 0121 248 2000
RoSPA provides information and advice on safety and accident prevention. Please send a stamped addressed envelope with any queries.

SCOPE (formerly the Spastics Society)
6 Market Road
London N7 9PW
Tel: 0171 619 7100
Helpline tel: 0800 626216 (11.00 am–9.00 pm Monday–Friday; 2.00 pm–6.00 pm weekends)
Website: http://www.scope.org.uk
SCOPE provides information and counselling service on cerebral palsy and associated disabilities. It manages a number of schools, education centres, units and residential centres for people with cerebral palsy.

SKILL (National Bureau for Students with Disabilities)
336 Brixton Road
London SW9 7AA
Tel: 0171 274 0565
Information line tel: 0171 978 9890 (1.30 pm–4.30 pm Monday–Friday)
email: skillnatburdis@compuserve.com
SKILL provides an information service for students with disabilities.

SOS Talisman
Talman Ltd
21 Grays Corner
Ley Street
Ilford
Essex IG2 7RQ
Tel: 0181 554 5579
SOS Talisman sells medical identification bracelets and necklaces.

SPOD (Association to aid the Sexual and Personal Relationships of
People with a Disability)
286 Camden Road
London N7 0BJ
Tel: 0171 607 8851
SPOD provides information and advice on the problems in sex and
personal relationships which disability can cause.

Tuberous Sclerosis Association
Little Barnsley Farm
Catshill
Bromsgrove
Worcestershire B61 0NQ
Tel: 01527 871898
email: tsassn@compuserve.com
Tuberous Sclerosis Association organizes meetings and conferences for
families and professionals. Provides financial help for families, research
and special clinics.

Appendix 2
Useful publications

At the time of writing, all the publications listed here were available. Those available through the British Epilepsy Association (address in Appendix 1) are marked with an asterisk. Check with them, the publishers or your local bookshop for current prices.

About epilepsy

General titles

* *Encyclopaedia of epilepsy* edited by David Chadwick, published by Roby Education (1997)

Epilepsy – A parent's guide by Joe McMenamin and Mary O'Connor Bird, published by Brainwave, The Irish Epilepsy Association (1993)

Epilepsy: the facts by Anthony Hopkins and Richard Appleton, published by Oxford University Press (1996)

* *Living with epilepsy – a practical guide to coping, causes and treatment* by David Chadwick and Sue Usiskin, published by Vermilion (1997)

Living with epilepsy: a guide to taking control by Dr Peter Fenwick and Elizabeth Fenwick, published by Bloomsbury (1996)

* *Your child's epilepsy* by Richard Appleton, Brian Chappell and Margaret Beirne, published by Class Publishing (1997)

Publications for children

Independence – epilepsy in teenagers by Richard Appleton and David Chadwick, published by Hoechst Marion Roussel (1996)

Magazines

* *Epilepsy Today*, published quarterly by the British Epilepsy Association

* *International Epilepsy News*, published quarterly by the International Bureau for Epilepsy (available in the UK through the British Epilepsy Association)

Books for professionals

Epilepsy edited by Anthony Hopkins, Simon Shorvon and Gregory Cascino, published by Chapman and Hall (2nd edition 1995)

Other publications

The various epilepsy associations publish a wide range of leaflets, booklets and videos on epilepsy. Write to them at the addresses in Appendix 1 for further details and a current price list.

Publications on other topics

HEA guide to complementary medicine and therapies by Anne Woodham, published by the Health Education Authority (1994)

Special educational needs – a guide for parents, published by the Department for Education and Employment (single copies in various languages free on request by writing to the DEE Publications Centre, PO Box 2193, London E15 2EU or by telephoning 0181 533 2000)

Taking a break, published by the King's Fund Carers Unit (single copies free to carers available from Taking a Break, Newcastle-upon-Tyne X, NE85 2AQ)

Traveller's guide to health, published by the Department of Health (single copies free on request by calling Freefone 0800 555 777)

Index

NOTE: this index is arranged alphabetically in letter by letter order covering pages 1 to 162. Page numbers in italics refer to tables or diagrams. Numbers followed by 'g' indicate glossary.

Have you found **Epilepsy at your fingertips** practical and useful? If so, you may be interested in other books from Class Publishing.

Heart health at your fingertips
NEW! £14.99
Dr Graham Jackson

Everything you need to know to keep your heart healthy – and live life to the full! This practical handbook, written by a leading cardiologist, answers all your questions about heart conditions

High blood pressure at your fingertips £14.99
Dr Julian Tudor Hart

The author uses all his 26 years of experience as a General Practitioner and blood pressure expert to answer your questions on high blood pressure.

Diabetes at your fingertips
FOURTH EDITION £14.99
Professor Peter Sönksen,
Dr Charles Fox and Sister Sue Judd

461 questions on diabetes are answered clearly and accurately – the ideal reference book for everyone with diabetes

'I will certainly recommend it to my patients ... I think it is brilliant.'
Robert Tattersall, Professor of Clinical Diabetes, Queen's Medical Centre, Nottingham

Parkinson's at your fingertips
£14.99
Dr Marie Oxtoby and
Professor Adrian Williams

Full of practical help and advice for people with Parkinson's disease and their families. This book gives you the information and the confidence to tackle the challenges that PD presents.

Allergies at your fingertips
NEW! £14.99
Dr Joanne Clough

At last – sensible, practical advice on allergies from an experienced expert.

'Extremely enjoyable and informative.'
Susan Ollier BSc, Scientific Director, British Allergy Foundation

Your child's epilepsy: a parent's guide £11.99
Dr Richard Appleton, Brian Chappell and Margaret Beirne

If your child has epilepsy, you will find this practical guide invaluable. It answers the questions you really want to ask from diagnosis to treatment, and from schools to relationships.

Stop that heart attack!
NEW!! £14.99
Dr Derrick Cutting

The easy, drug-free and medically *accurate* way to cut your risk of suffering a heart attack dramatically.
Don't be a victim – take action now!

Alzheimer's at your fingertips
NEW! £14.99
Harry Cayton, Dr Nori Graham,
Dr James Warner

At last – a book that tells you everything you need to know about Alzheimer's and other dementias.

'an invaluable contribution to understanding all forms of dementia.'
Dr Jonathan Miller CBE, President of the Alzheimer's Disease Society

Cancer information at your fingertips
NEW SECOND EDITION £14.99
Val Speechley and Maxine Rosenfield

Recommended by the Cancer Research Campaign, this books provides straightforward, practical and positive answers to all your questions about cancer.

Asthma at your fingertips
NEW SECOND EDITION   £14.99
Dr Mark Levy, Professor Sean Hilton and
Greta Barnes MBE

This book shows you how to keep your
asthma – or your family's asthma – under
control, making it easier to live a full,
happy and healthy life.

> 'This book gives you the knowledge. Don't
> limit yourself.'
> *Adrian Moorhouse, MBE,*
> *Olympic Gold Medallist*

PRIORITY ORDER FORM

Cut out or photocopy this form and send it (post free in the UK) to:

Class Publishing Customer Service   Tel: 01752 202301
FREEPOST (no stamp needed)
LONDON W6 7BR   Fax: 01752 202333

		Post included price per copy
Please send me urgently (tick boxes below)		**(UK only)**

☐	**Epilepsy at your fingertips** (ISBN 1 872362 51 6)	£17.99
☐	**Heart health at your fingertips** (ISBN 1 872362 77 X)	£17.99
☐	**High blood pressure at your fingertips** (ISBN 1 872362 48 6)	£17.99
☐	**Diabetes at your fingertips** (ISBN 1 872362 79 6)	£17.99
☐	**Parkinson's at your fingertips** (ISBN 1 872362 47 8)	£17.99
☐	**Allergies at your fingertips** (ISBN 1 872362 52 4)	£17.99
☐	**Your child's epilepsy: a parent's guide** (ISBN 1 872362 61 3)	£17.99
☐	**Stop that heart attack!** (ISBN 1 872362 85 0)	£17.99
☐	**Alzheimer's at your fingertips** (ISBN 1 872362 71 0)	£17.99
☐	**Cancer information at your fingertips** (ISBN 1 872362 56 7)	£17.99
☐	**Asthma at your fingertips** (ISBN 1 872362 67 2)	£17.99

TOTAL: _____

Easy ways to pay

Cheque: I enclose a cheque payable to Class Publishing for £_____

Credit card: please debit my ☐ Access ☐ Visa ☐ Amex ☐ Switch

Number: _____ Expiry date: _____

Name _____

My address for delivery is _____

_____

Town _____ County _____ Postcode _____

Telephone number (in case of query) _____

Credit card billing address if different from above _____

_____

Town _____ County _____ Postcode _____

Class Publishing's guarantee: remember that if, for any reason, you are not satisfied with these books, we will refund all your money, without any questions asked. Prices and VAT rates may be altered for reasons beyond our control.